Praise for *A Baby at Last!*

"One of my   loving wife,
Bernadette.   oldstein. He
is the best 'c   y Olympic
gold medal, r   anks due to
Dr. Goldsteir

rld Champion

"A clear and   rt diagnosis
and treatmen   oth authors
are world re   fer sensible
advice and g   ies of male
and female f   ironmental,
and emotiona   ommend to
the couple sta

Making Babies:
imum Fertility

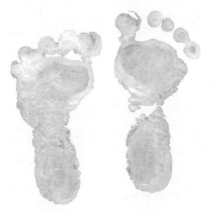

A Baby at Last!

The Couple's Complete Guide to Getting Pregnant—
from Cutting-edge Treatments to Commonsense Wisdom

Zev Rosenwaks, M.D., and Marc Goldstein, M.D.,
OF THE WEILL CORNELL MEDICAL COLLEGE OF CORNELL UNIVERSITY,

and Mark L. Fuerst

A Fireside Book
PUBLISHED BY SIMON & SCHUSTER
NEW YORK LONDON TORONTO SYDNEY

Fireside
A Division of Simon & Schuster, Inc.
1230 Avenue of the Americas
New York, NY 10020

The names and identifying details of some individuals have been changed.

First Fireside trade paperback edition June 2010

FIRESIDE and colophon are registered trademarks of Simon & Schuster, Inc.

For information about special discounts for bulk purchases,
please contact Simon & Schuster Special Sales at 1-866-506-1949
or business@simonandschuster.com.

The Simon & Schuster Speakers Bureau can bring authors to your live event.
For more information or to book an event contact the Simon & Schuster
Speakers Bureau at 1-866-248-3049 or visit our website at www.simonspeakers.com.

Designed by Ruth Lee-Mui

Manufactured in the United States of America

10   9   8   7   6   5   4   3   2   1

Library of Congress Cataloging-in-Publication Data

Rosenwaks, Zev.
   The couple's complete guide to getting pregnant from cutting-edge treatments to
commonsense wisdom / by Zev Rosenwaks, Marc Goldstein, and Mark L. Fuerst.
      p.   cm.
   "A Fireside Book."
   Includes bibliographical references and index.
   1. Infertility—Popular works.   2. Human reproductive technology—Popular works.
I. Goldstein, Marc.   II. Fuerst, Mark L.   III. Title.
   RC889.R843   2010
   616.6'92—dc22   2010009463

ISBN 978-1-4391-4962-1
ISBN 978-1-4391-7236-0 (ebook)

To Stacy, Barbara, and Margie,
and all the couples we have had the privilege of helping

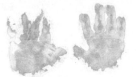

Acknowledgments

$\mathcal{M}$any people helped us in the long process of making this book a reality. We would like to thank the entire staff at the Center for Reproductive Medicine and Infertility for their help, with particular recognition to Carlene Mowl for her handling of the editorial and visual material that went into the preparation of the manuscript. We would also like to thank Vanessa Dudley for her invaluable help in preparation of the manuscript and creation of the medical illustrations, as well as the rest of the staff at the Center for Male Reproductive Medicine and Microsurgery at Weill Cornell for the fabulous care of our couples, and all the Weill Cornell Medical College residents and fellows whose assistance in the care of our patients and research has helped advance our field. We would also thank our agent, Linda Konner, for coming up with a great title and for her persistence and support throughout the project, our editor Michelle Howry and the staff at Simon & Schuster for putting it all together, and the Brooklyn Brown Bag Lunch Group for brainstorming and encouragement.

Contents

Part III. Advanced Technologies and Treatments

Introduction

*E*veryone seems to know someone who has a fertility problem, because infertility is really that pervasive. It's talked about more openly now, and new developments make headlines on the evening news and the covers of celebrity magazines. People chat on social-networking Web sites about their infertility. You may hear about a new procedure via an article you found on the Web or from others experiencing the same thing you are going through. You talk about the kinds of tests and treatments you receive and what combinations of drugs you are on. You are determined to find a way to have a baby.

Our program, honed over the last twenty years at Weill Cornell Medical Center, one of the top fertility clinics in the world, offers an approach to patient care that brings together all of the services that couples may need. What's different about us is our balanced approach to fertility treatments. We look not just at the female or just the male, but at you together as a couple. Whatever the problem may be, it is worked up, uncovered, and dealt with. Certain clues lead to male or female problems; we know how to recognize those clues.

Our couples-based fertility approach is surprisingly unique—and remarkably effective. Half of all women under age 35 going through one in vitro fertilization (IVF) cycle at Weill Cornell take home a baby. The Center for Reproductive Medicine and Infertility, run by Dr. Zen Rosenwaks, offers the most advanced fertility services you might need. The Center for Male Reproductive Medicine and Microsurgery, run by Dr. Marc Goldstein, was the first male infertility center established at a university medical center to collaborate with a comprehensive IVF program. To ensure that both women and men have access to the widest possible range of superior services, the two centers have joined to establish the Cornell Institute for Reproductive Medicine. Even if you can't get an appointment with us here at our clinic, we'll show you how to learn from our processes and achieve your dream—a baby at last.

We also run an intensive program of clinical and scientific research that has furthered the understanding of human reproduction and, most significantly, culminated in innovative ways to optimize fertility treatments. These cutting-edge clinical and technological capabilities, paired with our emphasis on treatment tailored to your individual, specific needs, have contributed to our success rates.

So Who Are We?

Dr. Rosenwaks is internationally known for his pioneering work in assisted reproduction. He was the director of the Jones Institute for Reproductive Medicine in Norfolk, Virginia, the unit that achieved the first IVF pregnancy in the United States. He also developed the first egg donation program in the United States. Dr. Rosenwaks and his team of female fertility specialists have helped more couples have babies through assisted reproduction than any other center in the country, and they have consistently achieved among the highest success rates in the world.

Dr. Goldstein is internationally renowned for his pioneering work in vasectomy reversals and microsurgical repair of varicoceles (varicose veins in the scrotum) and blockages. He developed a microsurgical technique of varicocele removal in 1984 and he was the first American surgeon to be trained in and perform the Chinese method of no-scalpel vasectomy.

For this book, we have relied upon the expertise of members of our fertility teams, who are among the most experienced and accomplished medical professionals in their fields, including specialists in reproductive endocrinology, reproductive urology, embryology, andrology, immunology, gynecology, and other related areas.

About *A Baby At Last!*

A Baby At Last! grew out of our closely associated clinical fertility practices at Weill Cornell, where, once a month, we hold combined male-fertility/female-fertility conferences to discuss our patients. Now we have put down on paper our expertise in a readable format for all couples facing infertility. The book shows, step by step, how we diagnose and treat the couples who come to us. If a couple is willing to take advantage of everything revealed in the book, from lifestyle changes to hormone treatments to surgery to state-of-the-art assisted reproductive technologies, it is likely that their infertility problem will resolve. And because infertility can affect couples in many ways, we offer advice on the emotional aspects of care, so you can better understand your treatment every step of the way.

In the book, we explain the most up-to-date therapies, many of them devised and perfected by Weill Cornell doctors. The book reflects our fertility practice by emphasizing the importance of evaluating and treating the couple together, not just the female or the male partner.

We break down the intricate science of what we do into simple language. Our own patients provide their stories in their own words of what it's like to go through what is often a rollercoaster ride of fertility treatments. In addition to introducing you to our successful fertility program, we also show you how to search fertility databases and compare programs and how to sort out what's on the Internet.

At the end of each chapter, we provide you with a short list of "Take Home Messages" to summarize what you've just learned. And at the end of most chapters you'll find new, still-experimental information that may be of interest in the near future.

Maybe you can't come to New York to consult with us directly. That's why we wrote this book: to offer you the information that has become known to the thousands of our patients who have had babies. Couples who follow the book's advice, along with their own doctor's help, can achieve the same amazing results we see every day in our own practices.

Reproductive medicine is an exciting, innovative field. Nothing is more rewarding to us than seeing our patients' dreams come true. Our goal in *A Baby At Last!* is to present to you the most effective, safest fertility treatments available—both the cutting-edge science and the surprisingly simple techniques. Then you and your doctors can tailor these treatments to meet your needs. We hope that you will find the information, insights, and specific treatments in the book that will help you comfortably complete your family and achieve your goal of having a baby at last.

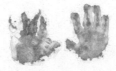

Part I

Getting Started on the Right Path

One

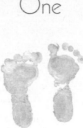

You Are Not Alone
When to Seek Help

· · · · · · · · · ·

Claire, a thirty-seven-year-old designer, had tried unsuccessfully to have a baby for a year and a half before she went to see her gynecologist. Her doctor found she had an incompetent cervix, which he corrected surgically. Six months later, her husband, Jeff, a thirty-eight-year-old salesman, went to a urologist, who found Jeff had a very low sperm count and a cyst on one testicle. Claire did some research on the Internet into hospitals and doctors. An oncologist friend suggested they go to Weill Cornell, where a radiologist told them that Jeff's cyst was benign, but Dr. Goldstein found that Jeff had varicoceles (varicose veins in the scrotum) affecting both testicles. Microsurgery repaired the varicoceles, but Jeff's sperm count remained very low, so they decided to try an in vitro fertilization (IVF) procedure with Dr. Rosenwaks.

For the first IVF attempt, three of Claire's eggs were fertilized with Jeff's sperm and transferred into her uterus, but none progressed to a pregnancy. A few months later, Jeff had better-quality sperm surgically removed from his testicles, and those sperm were used to fertilize ten of Claire's eggs. Dr. Rosenwaks transferred four healthy embryos.

"I had prepared myself for the possibility that it wouldn't work," says Claire. "Jeff and I talked a lot during the two-week wait about what we would do if we got bad news. We also met with a counselor at Weill Cornell, who made the process easier to deal with." When they received word that Claire was pregnant, "I

couldn't believe it," says Jeff. "I'll never forget that call." Their daughter, Connie, is now eighteen months old.

. . . .

Fertility is, on the face of things, a very simple process. It's a matter of getting the sperm and egg together. But the variables are plentiful, and as many couples find, it's easy for something to go wrong. You need a good-quality egg and properly functioning sperm. You need enough sperm to be deposited where it's supposed to be. The sperm has to be strong enough to swim up the female reproductive tract through the fallopian tube to reach the egg to fertilize it. The fallopian tube has to be normal to be able to pick up the fertilized egg and deliver it to the uterus so it can develop fully. The woman's brain also needs to function properly, so that the pituitary gland produces adequate amounts of hormones necessary to foster follicle and egg development in the ovary. In turn the ovary, under the influence of the pituitary gland, must produce the critical hormones—estrogen and progesterone—necessary to promote uterine lining development and support for the implantation of the fertilized egg.

This whole series of events needs to happen at the right time. There is an eight-to-twelve-hour window within each cycle in which the egg can become fertilized. Usually this happens between days 13 and 15 of a typical twenty-eight-day menstrual cycle. Healthy sperm can survive for several days inside the female reproductive tract, so timing sex around the middle of the cycle increases your chances of conception. Even in the best of circumstances, the chances that a woman will get pregnant are about one in four each month.

You Are Not Alone

There are many reasons a couple may find it hard to get pregnant, and these reasons can stem from a problem with either or both partners. In about 40 percent of infertile couples, the man has a problem. In another 40 percent, the woman has a problem. And in 20 percent *both* partners have a problem. That's why a couples-based solution is imperative.

Often both partners may have just-below-normal fertility, or subfertility, which may lead them to struggle with having a baby together. Treatments to improve each partner's fertility will maximize their chances of conceiving.

Many infertile couples striving to conceive feel isolated and helpless, but actually you are not alone. Infertility affects about 7 million Americans, which represents about one in six couples during their childbearing years. These are daunting odds, but here's the good news: while the number of infertile couples is on the rise, medical understanding of infertility is more advanced than ever. You have more treatment options today than before. Just a few decades ago, there were no drugs to induce ovulation, no microsurgical techniques to unclog fallopian tubes in women or blocked ducts in men, IVF was just a dream, and single-sperm injections were unheard-of. And our understanding of the nonsurgical methods of increasing fertility—diet, exercise, and other lifestyle adjustments that greatly increase the odds of conceiving—is now similarly advanced.

When to Seek Help

You may feel lots of anxiety and stress about making a baby, particularly if you have been trying for a while. So it is important to know when it is appropriate to seek advice regarding your infertility. Fertility declines rapidly after age thirty-five, so women in this age group should consider working with a fertility specialist sooner rather than later. Even if you became pregnant on your own when you were younger, you may still have difficulty conceiving when you become older.

We begin to be concerned about infertility when a couple has not conceived after twelve months of unprotected intercourse if the woman is under age thirty-five, and six months of unprotected intercourse if she is age thirty-five or older. However, our policy is to recommend an evaluation if the female partner is older than age thirty and has not conceived within six months, especially if the couple has been having sexual intercourse two or three times per week.

If you are over age thirty, or if you or your partner has reason to believe there is a risk factor in your background (such as a history of genital infections, irregular periods, or cancer treatment), this certainly justifies an early fertility evaluation. We also suggest that a woman who has a history of two or more miscarriages and no live births seek out a fertility specialist. If you and your partner are over age thirty or there are clues from your past that either one of you might have a fertility problem, and you still don't get pregnant after optimizing your chances by timing intercourse around ovulation, then we believe you need not wait as long as six months before seeking medical help.

If you and your partner have been trying to have a baby for about a year with no success, you may have fertility problems as a couple. But this does not mean you will never have a baby. Fertility problems are common and shared among men and women, and treatments are available. In fact, most of the couples who seek our help will eventually have a baby.

Fertility through the Decades

We are able to help young couples in their twenties who are having a difficult time achieving a pregnancy, couples in their thirties who may already have one child but can't seem to have another one, and even women into their forties and rarely in their fifties who thought having a baby was beyond their reach.

Most women know that it's harder to *get* pregnant when they get older. But complications *during* pregnancy also become more common with age. Age increases the risk of miscarriage and the need for a cesarean delivery and also increases the chances of pregnancy-related diabetes and of having twins.

At birth, a woman has all the eggs she will ever have. As she ages, so do her eggs. And as an egg ages, it is more likely to develop a chromosomal abnormality. A fertilized egg with abnormal chromosomes is the single most common cause of miscarriage; at least half of all miscarriages are due to abnormal chromosomes. A woman in her twenties has a 10 percent chance of having a miscarriage each time she becomes pregnant. In her late thirties, the odds of a miscarriage are about 20 percent to 30 percent because of declining egg quality, and a woman in her forties faces a 50 percent to 60 percent risk of miscarriage.

Although age has a significant impact on pregnancy outcome and infertility, advancing age alone should not prevent you from trying to become pregnant. More than one third of all pregnancies and births in the United States occur in women who are in their thirties or older. Good prenatal obstetrical care has made pregnancies in older women safer than they were twenty to thirty years ago. The following sections illustrate typical scenarios in couples achieving pregnancies at different decades of their reproductive life.

A Baby in Your Twenties

. . . .

Nan, age twenty-seven, and her husband, Brad, also twenty-seven, had struggled with infertility for several years. "I had a diagnosis of polycystic ovaries from my gynecologist, who started me on fertility pills. But they didn't work. I needed something more," says Nan. They went to see Dr. Rosenwaks, who suggested they try intrauterine insemination (IUI). Two months later, they began an IUI attempt, with Nan taking gonadotropin injections during her menstrual cycle. Nan became pregnant in that first IUI attempt. Their baby, Amy, is now seven months old "You think that if you just keep trying, it will happen. But if you have a problem, it's better to take care of it in a timely manner," says Nan.

. . . .

In 1970, American women typically had their first child at twenty-one. Today, most women are about twenty-five when they give birth. A woman in her twenties is likely to have healthier eggs than older women, which generally makes it easier to conceive. High-quality eggs also translate into a lower risk of birth defects. At twenty-five, the likelihood of having a baby with Down syndrome is about 1 in 1,250. Those with Down syndrome generally have one extra chromosome 21, for a total of forty-seven instead of the normal forty-six, and carrying a fetus with Down syndrome or another chromosomal disorder is often the reason women lose a pregnancy. This is one reason that miscarriage is less common in younger women. Younger women are also well equipped to handle the physical demands of pregnancy. But as many twenty-something women learn, fertility problems can arise at any age. The treatments in this book offer women in their twenties who are struggling to get pregnant the tools they need.

A Baby in Your Thirties

. . . .

After four years of trying, Donna, a thirty-seven-year-old store owner, had been unable to conceive with her husband, David, thirty-nine, an independent film-maker. "All my life I knew I wanted to be a mother," says Donna. Having seen four different doctors and spent tens of thousands of dollars on treatments, she feared that her time was running out.

Tests at Weill Cornell showed that Donna's eggs were healthy but that David's sperm count was very low. The only way Donna could get pregnant was through an injection of David's sperm directly into her eggs in the laboratory, a process called intracytoplasmic sperm injection (ICSI), and then to have the fertilized egg implanted into her uterus. The procedure was a success, and Donna and David now have a one-year-old son, Don.

. . . .

According to data from the National Center for Health Statistics, birth rates for women ages thirty-five to thirty-nine doubled between 1978 and 2000. In fact, 20 percent of women in the United States now have their first child after age thirty-five.

Having a baby in your early thirties is much like being pregnant in your twenties. Your health, energy, and fertility are still likely to be at high levels, and the quality of your eggs is still very good, making the risks of genetic defects low. However, once you reach age thirty-five, the risk of losing a pregnancy is higher. And once you turn thirty-five, your pregnancy should be monitored more closely because of the rising risk of birth defects. We offer all of our patients an amniocentesis and/or other screening tests to check for Down syndrome and other chromosomal abnormalities. There's no need to panic, because about 95 percent of women who undergo prenatal testing receive good news.

A Baby in Your Forties

. . . .

Nicky, a forty-year-old social worker, had been trying to become pregnant for two years without success. Her gynecologist was baffled. There was no good medical reason for Nicky's infertility. She was in good health and her husband Leon, a forty-nine-year-old lawyer, had an excellent sperm count.

After extensive tests, the Weill Cornell team told them they were among the group with "unexplained" infertility, and suggested they opt for IVF. Their first try failed, and so they tried again. This time the procedure worked, and Nicky gave birth to a girl, Olivia.

. . . .

Women in their forties are a lot healthier than they were even a generation ago, making pregnancy a viable—and achievable—option for these women. However, the risk of birth defects is a growing concern. Older eggs are more likely to have chromosomal abnormalities in their embryos. At age forty, the chances that a fetus will have Down syndrome is one in one hundred, and at age forty-five the chance is one in thirty. Due to these higher risks, it is essential that prenatal genetic tests be performed.

What's more, first-time mothers over forty are more likely to develop high blood pressure and diabetes during pregnancy than mothers in their twenties. And they are more likely to suffer placenta previa, a condition in which the placenta is implanted low in the uterus, which can impede delivery. This condition can cause complications, but these can often be prevented with a cesarean delivery.

If you're over forty and trying to conceive, you're in good company. Technological advances such as better IVF techniques now make it easier for women in their forties to have babies. With the extension of life expectancy for older women, the benefits of hormonal replacement therapy, and general improvement of the health and living conditions of older women, very late childbearing has become more socially acceptable. However, the chance of becoming pregnant with one's own eggs is very difficult after the age of forty-two or forty-three. Many women in this age group must turn to egg donation.

Some women who seek to conceive after age forty have no difficulty in achieving a pregnancy as long as they have a prompt, thorough evaluation and undergo aggressive treatments.

One simple blood test—measuring the level of follicle-stimulating hormone (FSH) in your blood on day 3 of your menstrual cycle—is important to assess the *ovarian reserve*, a term used to describe the number of eggs remaining in a woman's ovary. The pituitary gland produces FSH, which is responsible for the development each month of an ovarian follicle, which contains an egg. When the ovaries have very few eggs remaining, the pituitary gland senses this and begins to produce and release higher and higher amounts of FSH in an effort to stimulate the ovary. For example, women who have gone through menopause and have few or no eggs remaining in their ovaries have exceedingly high levels of FSH in their blood. Young women who have had an accelerated decline in the number of eggs can also have high FSH levels. FSH is probably more an indirect measure of egg quantity than an indicator of quality.

If the blood test shows that your FSH levels are consistently elevated, you have a much lower chance of conceiving and carrying to term; if your FSH levels are slightly above normal, these baseline levels suggest that you have a lower chance of achieving a pregnancy.

Other findings we associate with an age-related decline in fertility include a shorter or irregular menstrual cycle, symptoms of impending menopause, and low numbers of egg-carrying follicles in response to stimulation with hormones. If you have had previous surgery affecting your ovaries, such as the removal of an ovarian cyst or partial removal of ovarian tissue, that might also lead to an earlier loss of ovarian function.

In the last few years we have added another ovarian marker to help us assess the ovarian reserve. The hormone called anti–Müllerian hormone (AMH) is produced by an early stage of the developing egg-containing ovarian follicles. Very low levels of AMH denote poor ovarian reserve, whereas high levels suggest that the woman has many eggs remaining in her ovary.

Unfortunately, there are no treatments available that can turn back the clock on a woman's ovaries, but there are many treatment options that can greatly help you in your quest to have a child. We can prescribe fertility drugs to try to increase your chances of pregnancy. These powerful hormones can increase the number of eggs that develop in a given month and enhance the chance that at least one of them might be able to be fertilized and develop into a pregnancy.

The one consistently successful method to improve pregnancy rates in women with age-related infertility is through a donor egg. You may be a candidate to receive a donor egg if you are over age forty, have persistently high FSH levels at any age, respond poorly to fertility drugs at any age, or have poor-quality embryos after undergoing an IVF cycle.

Lots of Options

You never know where you will fall in the fertility lottery, so you may need to hedge your bets the best you can, particularly if you're in your late thirties or forties. You should probably talk with your doctor about donor-egg IVF, embryo development in the laboratory, and preimplantation genetic diagnosis (PGD).

Donor-Egg IVF

For some women, the only hope is to use donor eggs. In this process, another woman's eggs are fertilized, either with her husband's or a donor's sperm, and the resulting embryo is transferred to the woman's uterus, which has been prepared to receive the embryo. While IVF success rates go down drastically after age thirty-seven, the success of donor eggs remains high.

With egg donation, success rates are dependent on the age of the donor rather than the recipient. We achieve live birth rates that exceed 50 percent per procedure with donors between twenty-one and thirty-four years of age. The use of donated eggs has made it possible for couples to achieve pregnancies when all other methods have been exhausted.

Embryo Development in the Laboratory

Another important approach to improve the success rate of IVF is to optimize the laboratory conditions for early embryos. We have developed a method to co-culture embryos with certain helper cells to enhance the development of fertilized eggs and improve embryo quality.

Endometrial co-culture is a laboratory method that utilizes the mother's own uterine lining cells to enhance embryo quality. Simply stated, in a separate menstrual cycle one to two months before undergoing an IVF procedure, the woman undergoes a biopsy of her endometrial lining seven to ten days after ovulation. The cells are separated, grown in the laboratory, and frozen, later to be thawed during the subsequent IVF cycle. After her eggs are fertilized through IVF techniques, the embryos are grown on top of the mother's extracted cells. This provides a better environment for the embryos, especially for couples who have exhibited poor embryo quality in previous IVF cycles.

Co-culture is usually reserved for use in "poor prognosis" patients, particularly when other cycles have failed because of slow growth of the embryo. This method is not a "cure" for age-related IVF failures, but in properly selected couples, it has significantly improved embryo quality.

Preimplantation Genetic Diagnosis

IVF technology allows us to analyze the genetic makeup of embryos that are developing outside the body. We can now remove a single cell from the developing embryo without harm and analyze that embryo for specific genetic disorders (or flaws) that may exist in either or both parents. By removing one or two cells from the embryo, we can successfully screen for genetic diseases such as cystic fibrosis, sickle cell disease, and Tay-Sachs disease, among many other conditions. More than two hundred genetic diseases have been successfully analyzed in preimplantation embryos.

Embryos can also be sorted to avoid X-linked (sex-linked) disorders such as hemophilia, muscular dystrophy, and many others. We can also detect chromosomal abnormalities in couples who suffer from recurrent pregnancy losses as well as in women who have miscarriages due to too many or too few chromosomes. If you have a sex-linked disorder, we can identify the gender of the embryos to avoid transmission of these diseases.

New methods of genetic screening allow us to screen for multiple disorders at the same time. Future developments in this area will allow us not only to diagnose genetic problems better but to treat genetically related disorders.

For more detailed information on donor eggs, see Chapter 13, and for more on embryo co-culture and PGD, see Chapter 12.

In the Future

Egg Maturation in the Laboratory

During an IVF cycle, eggs are recovered from a woman's ovaries after a seven-to-twelve-day treatment with hormones to stimulate her ovaries. In this process we override the woman's natural tendency to produce a single egg. On average, we aim to harvest between five and fifteen eggs. These eggs are then fertilized with the male partner's sperm, and the ensuing embryos are then transferred into the woman's uterus.

Unfortunately, not all women respond to the stimulating hormones in a predictable fashion. Some respond excessively and others not at all. One potential approach to circumvent stimulation problems is to collect immature eggs and mature them in the laboratory. While this approach is not quite as effective as conventional IVF, it is being optimized in several laboratories throughout the world. This could be the treatment of choice for women when ovarian stimulation is not recommended for medical reasons.

Other approaches to optimizing IVF success include the detection of certain factors within the egg that are important for normal embryo development. These factors could reside in certain manufacturing structures within the egg itself or in the genetic material. Future developments may be able to replace specific missing factors that could overcome problems related to infertility.

Fertility on Ice

As more and more women delay childbearing, they are seeking ways to keep their fertility options open. Traditionally, these fertility preservation methods were made available to women who were facing radiation or chemotherapy and were likely to lose their reproductive function. Nowadays many women wish to preserve their future fertility for social reasons.

Embryo freezing is the most efficient and effective method of preserving fertility. This requires the woman to undergo ovarian stimulation, use her partner's or a donor's sperm to fertilize the eggs, and freeze the resulting embryos. However, many young women and girls do not have a partner and can only have eggs or ovarian tissue frozen.

Egg freezing is a potential way to save eggs for future use. Young women may eventually deposit high-quality eggs into a reproductive bank for use when they are older, just as men can freeze their sperm and place them in sperm banks. Later, when a woman is ready to have a baby, she can simply go to the bank and withdraw what she needs.

Mature eggs are notoriously tricky to freeze safely. Newer freezing media rely on higher concentrations of coolants and faster cooling times. This results in glasslike solutions rather than icelike frozen ones that can damage the egg. Even so, only a proportion of eggs survive thawing. Some babies have been born from thawed frozen eggs in women who cannot undergo ovarian stimulation, but this is still considered a largely experimental treatment.

. . . .

Technological advances such as these, along with ever-improving IVF techniques, make it possible for more women than ever before to have babies. You'll learn more about these fertility treatments as you read *A Baby at Last!* The first step to get you started on the right path is to figure out whether you or your partner is at risk for infertility, and you'll find help with this in Chapters 2 and 3.

Take-Home Messages

- If you are a woman over age thirty and have not conceived within six months of having unprotected sexual intercourse two to three times per week, you should have a fertility workup.
- Advancing age impacts a woman's fertility and pregnancy outcome but should not prevent you from trying to have a baby.
- Two of the most important tests to assess the number of eggs remaining in a woman's ovary are measurements of FSH in the blood on day 3 of the menstrual cycle, as well as AMH levels.

Two

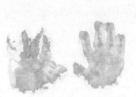

What Factors Determine His Fertility?
Risk Factors for Male Infertility

. . . .

After Ernie, age thirty-five, and Maude, age thirty-eight, had tried to conceive for one year with no luck, Maude went to her gynecologist. "We were both in our mid-thirties and didn't want to mess around if there was anything going on," says Ernie, an artist. "We did two intrauterine inseminations (artificial insemination directly into the uterine cavity) without success, so Maude's ob-gyn recommended I see Dr. Goldstein."

Ernie told Dr. Goldstein that as an adolescent he had an undescended right testicle. That testicle still rose up inside his abdomen whenever Ernie jogged or exercised. Dr. Goldstein noted that his right testicle was small in size and that he had a large varicocele (varicose vein in the scrotum) in his normally descended left testicle. Ernie's semen analysis showed a low sperm count and poor sperm morphology (structure). "Dr. Goldstein suggested an operation on both the undescended right testicle and the varicocele on the left side," recalls Ernie.

Dr. Goldstein correctly placed Ernie's right testicle into his scrotum and microsurgically repaired the varicocele in the left testicle. "We waited six months, and my sperm numbers improved, but we still needed to go to in vitro fertilization," says Ernie. At age forty, Maude, also an artist, became pregnant and delivered naturally at full term. Their son, Peter, is now two years old.

. . . .

Most fertility doctors and fertility books focus on the female side of the fertility equation. But we know this is only half the story. In our integrated male/female fertility practice, we address both partners' fertility at the same time, saving couples precious time and garnering better results.

What Factors Determine His Fertility?

A man's fertility depends on sperm quantity, quality, and swimming power (motility). Healthy, normally shaped sperm in a man's ejaculate have to be strong-enough swimmers to travel up through the fertile mucus produced by a woman's cervix to reach the uterus and then through the fallopian tubes to reach the egg.

Sperm Quantity

A man produces, on average, 127 million sperm per day. That's about 1,000 sperm per heartbeat. It takes about three months for fully functioning sperm to develop within the body. A man who has more than 20 million sperm per milliliter of semen and a total of more than 40 million sperm in the ejaculate is considered to be fertile. Only about two hundred to a thousand of the millions of sperm in the ejaculated semen actually make the trip through the woman's fallopian tube to reach the egg, and only one sperm gets to fertilize that egg.

Sperm Quality

The quality of a man's sperm is just as important as the number and total amount of sperm. Sperm shape and structure must be normal. A man is most likely to be fertile if 30 percent or more, using World Health Organization criteria, or 14 percent, using strict (or Kruger) criteria, of his sperm are of normal shape and structure. A normal sperm has an oval head and a long tail to propel it forward. Sperm with large, small, tapered, or crooked heads or curled, kinked, or double tails are less likely to fertilize an egg.

Sperm Motility

To reach the egg, a man's sperm have to be good swimmers. They learn how to swim in the epididymis, the two-inch-long coiled tube that sits on the back of each of the testicles. Sperm ride the semen wave and then swim the last few inches to reach the egg. A man is most likely to be fertile if at least 50 percent of his sperm move progressively forward.

Under the best of circumstances, only about half to three quarters of a man's sperm are healthy enough to fertilize an egg. The quality of a man's sperm varies from day to day and from one ejaculate to the next. A man may produce the same concentration of sperm but with a widely different volume of semen, sperm count, and motility. If these sperm values are just below normal, which is called subfertility, it may be that one or more of the following risk factors is the culprit.

Sperm can be especially vulnerable to certain medical conditions, medications taken for some very common illnesses such as heart disease and cancer, a lifestyle that includes smoking cigarettes and heavy use of alcohol or recreational drugs, and environmental factors such as exposure to chemicals, including pesticides. And while the biological clock certainly ticks for women, an older man's sperm count and quality may also be depleted.

Medical Conditions and Infertility

Many medical conditions are associated with male fertility. However, some specific conditions have dramatic effects, including diabetes, neurological problems, undescended testicles, genetic disorders (most prominently cystic fibrosis), and lupus, as well as some types of surgery.

Excess sugar in the body, one of the consequences of diabetes, has a direct effect on sperm quality. Diabetes causes DNA damage in sperm, which means that diabetes adversely influences male fertility at a molecular level. The DNA in the nuclei of the sperm cells has greater levels of fragmentation in diabetic men than in men without the disease. In diabetic men there may also be more deletions of DNA in the tiny, energy-generating structures in the cells called *mitochondria*.

DNA damage in sperm can impair male fertility and reproductive health. Poor sperm DNA quality is associated with decreased embryo quality, low embryo implantation rates, higher miscarriage rates, and some serious child-hood diseases, in particular some childhood cancers.

In addition, diabetics often have a decreased amount of fluid in their ejaculate and erection problems because of neurological damage. Diabetic neuropathy tends to be a slowly progressing condition. The first symptom is usually a decrease in the amount of the ejaculate. The semen volume continues to decrease further until a man achieves an orgasm without any visible ejaculate. Without treatment at an early stage, the nerve damage con-tinues, leading to erection problems.

Any condition that impairs spinal cord function, such as a traumatic injury to the spine or multiple sclerosis, can lead to ejaculation problems. If the nerves running from the back down to the testicles and the epididymis become damaged, this impedes ejaculation. Men with spinal cord injuries can have ejaculation that goes back into the bladder instead of coming out of the penis.

Cancers or any medical condition that requires chemotherapy or radia-tion therapy can affect male fertility. Chemotherapy associated with testicu-lar cancer and lymphoma causes significant and irreversible sperm damage in 25 percent of men. The more drugs are used in chemotherapy and the longer the treatment lasts, the greater the odds are against a man becoming fertile again.

The most frequent congenital birth defect in male children is an unde-scended testicle, or *cryptorchidism*. Men with one undescended testicle (uni-lateral cryptorchidism) have slightly lower fertility potential and tend to have lower sperm counts. Men with two undescended testicles (bilateral cryptorchidism) have markedly decreased sperm counts, and their fertil-ity potential is significantly reduced. A small percentage of men born with cryptorchidism are more likely to have genetic mutations, including Kline-felter syndrome, which is the most common genetic cause of male infertility and is present in one in every six hundred men.

In the past, males with undescended testicles did not have surgery to bring the testicle into the scrotum until age seven or eight years. Over the years, this surgery has been performed earlier—as early as the first year after birth. Early surgery may improve fertility potential, although other factors, such as the location and appearance of the testicles, may play a role in future fertility.

The most common genetic disorder identified through family history is cystic fibrosis. Most men with full-blown cystic fibrosis are infertile due to the absence of the vas deferens (sperm-carrying duct), but men with cystic fibrosis are living longer, and using new sperm extraction techniques plus IVF or IVF with ICSI, some have passed the gene along to their children. Other less common genetic disorders, such as androgen receptor deficiencies, polycystic kidney disease, and intersex conditions, may also cause male reproductive problems.

Sperm abnormalities have also been seen in male patients with systemic lupus erythematosis, otherwise know as lupus. Lupus is an autoimmune disease that mainly affects women in their reproductive years. Male lupus patients have been found to have a high frequency of sperm abnormalities, including lower sperm counts, motility, and volume, and lower percentages of normally formed sperm, associated with smaller testicle size. Frequent intravenous treatment with the immunosuppressant drug cyclophosphamide appears to damage these men's testicles.

Certain symptoms might lead you to suspect you have a fertility problem. Chronic pain in the testicles or scrotum may be associated with an underlying disorder such as a varicocele or testicular tumor, which can cause fertility problems. Painful ejaculations or blood in your semen may represent disorders of the prostate or the seminal vesicles. Typically, these symptoms are due to inflammatory conditions, but you may have a congenital problem that affects your fertility. A lack of sense of smell is typically associated with Kallmann syndrome, a specific genetic variant of hypogonadotropic hypogonadism. The brain's hypothalamus does not produce gonadotropin-releasing hormone that normally stimulates the pituitary gland to put out the hormones LH and FSH, which in turn stimulate the testicles to make testosterone and sperm.

Several types of surgery can affect fertility. Surgery in the pelvic or abdominal area can affect the nerves that control erection and ejaculation. Hernia surgery can damage either the blood supply to the testicles or the vas deferens. Damage is often related to a restricted blood supply rather than direct damage to the vas deferens, and therefore may not be recognized at the time of surgery. Late scarring from an inflammatory reaction can also obstruct these tiny sperm-carrying tubes. Any kind of surgery near the scrotum, such as hydrocele surgery, can obstruct or scar the vas deferens or epididymis, the sperm-carrying tubes. Therefore we recommend that men of reproductive age not undergo scrotal or hernia surgery without informing the surgeon of their need for future fertility.

Contracting mumps as an adolescent or an adult as well as trauma to the testicles from an accident, a fall, or playing sports may also damage sperm production.

Medications

Many common prescription medications are well known to affect a man's fertility. The ulcer drug cimetidine (Tagamet) can increase estrogen levels and depress normal sperm formation. The inflammatory bowel disease drug sulfasalazine (Azulfidine) causes low sperm counts, decreases sperm motility, and increases the number of abnormally shaped sperm. Many antibiotics, including nitrofurantoin (Furadantin), which is used to treat urinary tract infections, inhibit sperm formation. The blood pressure and heart drug propranolol (Inderal) impairs sperm motility. Calcium channel blockers such as nifedipine (Procardia) and diltiazem (Cardizem) interfere with the chemical change that enables sperm to penetrate the egg. The antigout drug colchicine may lead to a zero sperm count.

Drugs That Affect Male Fertility

Prescription Drugs	Recreational Drugs
Cimetidine (Tagamet)	Alcohol
Sulfasalazine (Azulfidine)	Marijuana
Nitrofurantoin (Furadantin)	Cocaine
Propranolol (Inderal)	Amphetamines
All calcium blockers, such as nifedipine (Procardia) and diltiazem (Cardizem)	
Colchicine	
Prazosin (Minipress)	
All SSRIs, such as fluoxetine (Prozac) and paroxetine (Paxil)	
Finasteride (Propecia and Proscar)	

Many medications contribute to ejaculation problems. Several categories of antidepressants, including monoamine oxidase inhibitors, selective serotonin reuptake inhibitors (SSRIs), and tricyclic antidepressants, as well as antipsychotics and benzodiazopines, typically cause a lack of orgasm. Other agents such as alpha blockers, which include many blood pressure and heart drugs including prazosin (Minipress) and thiazides, may cause either retrograde ejaculation or no ejaculation.

Antidepressants such as fluoxetine (Prozac) and other SSRIs may make you feel better but may affect your sexual health. The use of SSRIs is one of the most common causes of delayed or missing ejaculation. In fact, SSRIs are intentionally used for men who have problems with too-early ejaculation. Prozac may also lead to decreased sex drive and to a lesser extent to impotence. In clinical studies that documented side effects of Prozac, a decreased sex drive occurred in up to 11 percent and impotence in up to 7 percent of those taking Prozac. SSRI-related sexual side effects usually disappear two to three weeks after discontinuing the medication.

Another SSRI, paroxetine (Paxil), seems to increase DNA fragmentation (small breaks in the chromosomes) in sperm. DNA integrity is crucial to normal fertility. Increased DNA fragmentation of sperm increases the risk of failure of intrauterine insemination. A large proportion of patients on SSRIs may have their fertility affected. The sperm of infertile men who take these drugs appears to be damaged by an unusual mechanism that slows down their transport through the body. Slowing down sperm transport can allow sperm to be damaged by higher temperatures or to be ejaculated after they should have been, that is, when they are too old. In some severe cases, the sperm are slowed down so much that almost no sperm appear in the ejaculate. A standard semen analysis won't measure all of these possible effects. A special test for DNA fragmentation may be needed for men taking this drug.

Antiandrogens, which are used to treat prostate enlargement and cancer, interfere with sperm production. Similarly, testosterone supplements also suppress sperm production. The brain senses the testosterone and sends a signal to the testicles to turn off testosterone production. This shuts down sperm production as well.

Men who use hair replacement drugs such as finasteride (Propecia) may unwittingly lower their fertility potential. Taking Propecia pills to treat male-pattern baldness may lead to potential side effects, including erectile dysfunction and impotence. A small percentage of men who use the standard 1 milligram daily dose of the drug report that they suffer erectile dysfunction, decreased semen volume, low libido, and breast tenderness and enlargement. These side effects are considered reversible and generally disappear within weeks when men discontinue using the drug. But men who discontinue the drug usually lose any hair they may have regrown, since the drug needs to be taken indefinitely to maintain hair growth and thickness.

Lifestyle Factors

A number of lifestyle factors play a role in a man's fertility, including smoking cigarettes, heavy drinking, stress, excessive weight, exposure to heat, recreational drug use, sexually transmitted diseases, genital infections that lead to sperm busters called antisperm antibodies, drugs to improve sexual performance, and even seemingly good-for-you health kicks.

Smoking

It's now well established that smoking cigarettes can have a negative impact on a man's sexual health. Smoking can, of course, affect lung capacity, heart health, and general vascular disease. Inevitably that also directly and indirectly adversely affects sexual and reproductive health.

Numerous reports and studies have confirmed that smoking reduces the quality and quantity of sperm. The key indicators of sperm quality are drastically reduced in men who smoke. Men who smoke cigarettes have lower sperm count, lower sperm motility, and increased abnormalities in sperm shape and function. Male smokers have an increase in dead and malformed sperm. Smoking also interferes with the adhesion of the sperm to the egg, which is vital for fertilization.

What's more, cigarette smoke can genetically damage sperm. Cigarette smoke is toxic to the genetic makeup of all cells but has a particularly negative effect on sperm, since sperm have no way of repairing damage to their genetic material. Smoking appears to generate free-radical damage to the DNA in sperm. This may explain the higher miscarriage rates among couples when the male partner smokes.

Other reports have found that men who smoke have lower sex drives and less frequent sex than nonsmokers. In addition, because the mechanism of developing an erection is dependent on healthy penile arteries and veins, smoking can also lead to impotence by causing damage to blood vessels. Smoking results in a buildup of fatty deposits in the arteries, which in turn block the flow of blood into the penis. And nicotine stimulation in the brain is thought to cause rapid contractions in penile tissue, again restricting blood flow through arteries. Finally, of course, it would be tragic to help a couple conceive and then have the father die prematurely of lung cancer or another smoking-related disease. The good news is that most smoking-related health issues can be reversed if the man stops smoking.

Heavy Drinking

Heavy drinking can take a toll on a man's reproductive health. Alcoholic men can develop signs of low testosterone, including shrunken testicles and enlarged breasts. Couples may have a higher risk of miscarriage if the man consumes ten or more drinks a week around the time of conception.

Problem drinking may dampen both a man's sex life and his chances of having children. Alcoholics tend to have lower testosterone levels and more sperm abnormalities than nondrinkers. They also have a far higher rate of erectile dysfunction.

Alcohol apparently enters the testicles directly, cuts testosterone production, and harms the quality of semen. It also interferes with the body's ability to absorb zinc from food, and zinc is a key mineral for male fertility.

On the bright side, it's unlikely that light drinking has any significant effect on a man's fertility.

Stress

Healthy sperm production depends on a complex balance and interaction of hormones. Any disruption in this process can hinder a couple's chances of conceiving. Chronic stress, whether it's from dealing with difficulties at work, financial worries, or family problems, can play havoc with a man's reproductive system.

Stress can lower the quality of a man's sperm, including the number of sperm and their swimming ability and shape, and lower his semen volume. Stress can affect the functioning of the hypothalamus, which is the gland in the brain that regulates the hormones required to produce testosterone. Stress has been linked to depressed testosterone levels.

Stress also can hurt a healthy sexual relationship and lead to loss of sex drive. Having sex less often means fewer chances to conceive.

Excessive Weight

An excess of body weight may reduce sperm concentration and sperm count, alter the delicate balance of sex hormones, and increase the temperature in the scrotum. Overweight men may also have lower libidos and have less sex than normal weight men, and may be at increased risk of erectile dysfunction.

Overweight men who have a body mass index (BMI) above 25 have lower volumes of seminal fluid and lower sperm counts than those with a BMI below 25, and also a higher proportion of abnormal sperm. Studies have also suggested an association between male obesity and increased DNA damage in the sperm, which can be associated with reduced fertility. You can calculate your BMI by multiplying your weight in pounds by 703 and then dividing the product by the square of your height in inches.

Compared with their thinner counterparts, obese men who have a BMI over 30 tend to have lower levels of testosterone in their blood, as well as lower levels of luteinizing hormone (LH) and follicle-stimulating hormone (FSH), which are both essential to reproduction. LH causes the testicles to produce sex hormones, and FSH stimulates sperm production. Excess body fat may increase the conversion of testosterone to estrogen in a man's blood. These hormone alterations could in turn signal the brain to suppress LH and FSH production.

Simple overheating of the testicles caused by excessive fat in the pelvic area may also contribute to fertility problems.

Heat Exposure

Sperm production is particularly sensitive to heat. Normal sperm production requires a testicular temperature that is slightly below the body's core temperature. Even a small additional heating effect on testicular temperature might be enough to affect a man's sperm quality. For example, men who regularly take hot baths, sit in hot tubs or Jacuzzis, or wear tight leather pants can raise the temperature of their testicles enough to impair their semen quality.

Sitting for ninety minutes on a heated seat found in some luxury cars or with a laptop computer on your lap may also be problematic. These seemingly innocuous activities may temporarily increase scrotal temperature and over time could affect a man's fertility.

Recreational Drugs

Recreational drugs, such as marijuana, cocaine, and amphetamines, and also anabolic steroids used for body building, have been implicated in male infertility, sometimes irreversibly.

Marijuana can decrease sperm density and motility and increase the number of abnormal sperm. Marijuana tends to upset hormone levels as well. Most of these effects are reversible by stopping smoking, but men who smoke too much marijuana may end up with irreversible damage. Cocaine can contribute to erectile dysfunction, and amphetamines can decrease sex drive.

Anabolic steroids, such as testosterone and its potent derivatives usually taken illegally, can shrink the testicles and drastically reduce fertility. Anabolic steroids are among the most dangerous group of legal prescription drugs besides the poisonous chemicals used to treat cancer. These drugs are widely available through an underground black market, mostly through weight-lifting gyms. But even in suburban health clubs, the denizens of the weight room know where to find steroids.

One of the more serious side effects of anabolic steroids is on male reproductive organs. Because of the high level of circulating testosterone caused by the steroids, the testicles no longer need to manufacture this hormone, so they begin to shrink. This reduces sperm production and may lead to both impotence and sterility.

Sexually Transmitted Diseases

A wide variety of sexually transmitted diseases (STDs), if left untreated, can scar and damage the epididymis, vas deferens, and ejaculatory ducts. Just one infection with an STD can partially or totally block the epididymis, and the chances of blockage increase with each STD episode.

The sheer volume of STDs is staggering. Up to half the U.S. population will acquire an STD by age thirty-five. Each year, the federal government's Centers for Disease Control and Prevention receive reports of about 2 million STDs, but population studies suggest that this is less than 40 percent of the actual cases. Estimates for new cases of gonorrhea exceed 600,000 per year, with more than 4 million new cases per year for infection with *Chlamydia trachomatis.*

A chlamydial infection may cause a burning sensation during urination and a puslike discharge from the penis within a week of infection. But up to 25 percent of men infected with chlamydia have no symptoms at all. About half of the men with nongonococcal urethritis (NGU), that is, inflammation of the urethra not due to gonorrhea, and almost half of those with acute infections of the epididymis, are infected with chlamydia. Inflammation of the urethra leads to the presence of white blood cells in the semen, which has been documented to impair sperm quality and function.

What's more, almost two thirds of men have not one but two genital infections, putting a double whammy on their reproductive tracts. Up to 40 percent of men with urethritis caused by gonorrhea also have an accompanying chlamydial infection.

Other organisms, including *Mycoplasma hominis* and a related organism, *Ureaplasma urealyticum,* can also cause urethritis and may impair sperm motility and fertilizing ability. Still other agents that cause urethritis include viruses, such as genital herpes simplex virus and human papilloma virus, and the protozoan *Trichomonas vaginalis.*

The human immunodeficiency virus (HIV) also seems to have a direct effect on fertility. HIV-positive men have been shown to have lower sperm counts and sperm motility compared with fertile noninfected men. Infected men also have a higher incidence of impaired sperm formation and smaller testicles. And long-term HIV-positive men have a fiftyfold greater risk of developing testicular cancer than the general population.

Sperm Busters

A genital tract infection can lead to the development of sperm busters known as antisperm antibodies. Antibodies are blood proteins made by the immune system's white blood cells to protect the body against invaders. Once it has identified an invader, the immune system produces a specific antibody to help the white blood cells fight it off. Sometimes the immune system recognizes a man's own sperm as foreign, similar to an infection, and produces antisperm antibodies against them.

How does this happen? Sperm are not produced until puberty, long after the body has learned to discriminate what is "self." Because the male genital tract is basically a closed tube, sperm are sequestered from the immune system. However, if the integrity of the male genital tract is breached and sperm leak out, then the sperm are viewed by the immune system as foreign. That's when the immune system responds by producing antibodies against the sperm.

Sperm can come into contact with a man's own blood or fluids in tissues due to trauma to the testicles, a weakness in the epididymis or vas deferens, a vasectomy (which deliberately severs the vas deferens), or a genital tract infection. Sperm placement outside the genital tract during anal intercourse is a risk factor for a woman developing antisperm antibodies or for a bisexual male. Men with cystic fibrosis, whose sperm-carrying tubes are missing, may also develop antisperm antibodies. Twisting of the testicles, called torsion, can damage them and lead to antisperm antibody production. In fact, about 5 percent of infertility is related to antisperm antibodies.

Antisperm antibodies can attach to a sperm's surface and alter the sperm's ability to fertilize eggs. They may prevent sperm from penetrating through cervical mucus if they are attached to a sperm's tail or may bar sperm from attaching to the egg or penetrating it if they are attached to the sperm's head. Also, antisperm antibodies on sperm can activate the immune system in the female genital tract and increase the likelihood that a woman will produce antisperm antibodies. Then her antisperm antibodies can impede sperm and prevent fertilization.

Where the antisperm antibodies are located in the body and how many there are determine how damaging they may be. Antibodies attached to sperm cause more male fertility problems than antibodies circulating in the blood. If less than half of a man's sperm have antibodies attached and the rest of the sperm are normal, then his chances of conception are good.

Sexual Enhancers

Young, healthy men are increasingly using sildenafil (Viagra) and other similar drugs recreationally as sexual enhancers; these drugs are not used just by older men who have erectile dysfunction. Young men need to know that the use of Viagra may adversely affect their sperm function and possibly their fertility.

There's both good and bad news about Viagra. Laboratory tests show that the drug leads to a sustained enhancement in numbers of progressively swimming sperm and their velocity. However, the amount of Viagra at concentrations equivalent to what a man would have thirty minutes after taking the maximum recommended 100 milligram dose leads to early activation of the acrosome reaction. The acrosome is the packet of enzymes in the sperm's head that produces enzymes to facilitate penetration of the egg. The acrosome reaction is the chemical change that enables a sperm to penetrate an egg. If sperm undergo the acrosome reaction too early, before they contact the egg, they are incapable of fertilization. So if the majority of sperm undergo the acrosome reaction on exposure to Viagra, the drug may significantly impair their fertilizing potential.

Young men who use these pills regularly, either recreationally or for erectile dysfunction, should undergo a complete health check, including a hormonal evaluation. Erectile dysfunction may be a symptom of underlying health issues, such as heart disease or diabetes, as well as low testosterone levels.

Health Kicks

Being in poor health can decrease a man's sperm production, but men who are too concerned with their health may also face problems. Heavy-duty workouts and very-low-fat or strict vegetarian diets may impair fertility.

Men who exercise to exhaustion may experience changes in their hormone levels and a drop in sperm count, sperm concentration, and semen volume. Interactions among the brain, the pituitary gland, and the testicles control fertility, and too much exercise could disrupt this hormone flow. This, in turn, affects sperm production.

Strenuous exercise—that is, training hard almost every day—may impair a man's fertility. Long-distance runners who go more than a hundred miles a week show reduced testosterone levels and lower sperm counts. More moderate exercise—running up to thirty-five miles a week—causes a slight drop in testosterone levels and a slight lowering of sperm counts.

A man who starts a low-calorie diet along with a vigorous exercise program to reduce his weight may also reduce his testosterone level. A diet that consists of a fat content of about 10 percent places a man at risk of having low testosterone levels. A strict vegetarian diet may also lead to infertility due to a zinc deficiency, since a man needs a sufficient amount of zinc to be able to produce sperm.

Environmental Impact

Exposure to chemicals such as pesticides in the water and ozone in the air seems to play a role in male infertility. The evidence is growing that chemicals in the environment affect both a man's sperm count and quality. Environmental factors seem to contribute to the severity of infertility and may worsen the effects of preexisting genetic or medical risk factors.

A range of pesticide classes has been investigated in male infertility, including pyrethroids, organophosphates, phenoxyacetic acids, carbamates, organochlorines, and pesticide mixtures. Studies have found an association between exposure to pesticides and low semen quality, DNA damage to sperm, and chromosome abnormalities. Pesticides have been shown to be responsible for men in rural areas having lower sperm counts and less vigorous sperm than men in urban areas. Also, men exposed to pesticides may have higher levels of the female hormone estradiol in their blood, and those exposed to solvents may have lower LH concentrations than nonexposed men. Besides direct exposure to pesticides, these chemicals leach into the ground water and end up in the water we drink.

Male reproductive function might be associated with exposure to polycyclic aromatic hydrocarbons (PAHs), which are widely found in our environment. PAHs are a group of more than one hundred chemicals that are formed by the incomplete combustion of coal, oil, wood, tobacco, charcoal-broiled meats, garbage, or other organic materials. The main sources of PAH emissions into the air are oil refineries, coal-tar production plants, paper mills, wood products manufacturers, aluminum production plants, and industrial machinery manufacturers. PAHs are also created in wood-burning stoves, fireplaces, indoor or outdoor grills, and the exhaust from automobiles. Some PAHs are found in medicines, dyes, plastics, pesticides, and wood preservatives. These chemicals can enter the body if we breathe in contaminated air, or consume contaminated food or water.

Researchers at Nanjing Medical University in China have found that high levels of PAHs in the urine place men at a higher risk for unexplained infertility. They found that men who have PAHs in their urine and also have abnormal semen quality (based on their semen volume, sperm concentration, sperm count, and sperm motility) may be at even higher risk for unexplained infertility.

There also appears to be a relationship between levels of atmospheric ozone and sperm development. Exposure to increased ozone levels in the air adversely affects developing sperm, leading to lower sperm quality. Ozone exposure may induce either an inflammatory reaction in the male genital tract or the formation of circulating toxic chemicals, both of which can cause a decline in sperm concentration.

The hormones in beef consumed by a pregnant woman might affect the future fertility of her son. Hormones such as estradiol, progesterone, testosterone, and anabolic steroids continue to be used as growth promoters in cattle. Residues of these chemicals remain in the meat after slaughter. University of Rochester researchers found that pregnant women who ate beef more than once a day had sons whose sperm counts were about 25 percent lower than in sons of women who ate beef less often. What's more, the sons of high beef consumers were more likely to have subfertile sperm counts. The men's own beef consumption did not have an impact on their sperm quality.

It's certainly true that chemicals in the environment may impact a man's reproductive health. The extent of the impact still remains an open question. For example, polychlorinated biphenyls (PCBs), synthetic organic chemicals that are used in hundreds of products, and phthalates, present in plastic food wrap, plastic tubing, and many over-the-counter products, do damage sperm. Men who are exposed to higher levels of PCBs have more damage to sperm DNA, which justifies concerns about PCB levels. But the amount of sperm with affected DNA is generally low, about 10 percent. The probability of fathering a child starts to decrease when the proportion of damaged sperm reaches about 20 percent. So PCB exposure might negatively impact a man's reproductive capabilities if he already has defective sperm for other reasons.

Most harmful products introduced into the environment get there without us knowing it. We have no control over this, and so it is very hard to avoid them. However, your genetic makeup and a healthy lifestyle may be able to neutralize or counterbalance the effects of pollutants. You'll find ways in Chapter 4 to help you take control of your reproductive health by living a healthier lifestyle.

Aging

Accumulating evidence now shows that a man's age is also an important factor in age-related infertility. Of course, male fertility does not drop as rapidly and permanently as female fertility. After all, Abraham was ninety-nine when his wife Sara became pregnant. We hear about May-December celebrity babies all the time. Yet all men gradually experience a condition called "andropause." Beginning in his thirties, a man's semen volume, sperm counts, and testosterone levels tend gradually to decrease. Men over the age of thirty-five have a steadily increasing number of genetically defective sperm and more fragmentation of sperm DNA. The incidence of varicoceles increases with age and men with varicoceles that were not repaired when they were younger experience an even more accelerated decline in testicular function.

Until recently there has been little clinical proof that simply being an older man has a direct effect on a couple's fertility. In a large study of couples undergoing IUI, French researchers found that couples where either the mother or the father was above age thirty-five had lower pregnancy rates. Perhaps more surprisingly, miscarriage rates also increased when the father was over age thirty-five. The researchers believe the culprit is damaged sperm DNA, which does increase with age.

The researchers in Paris suggest that infertile couples where either partner is above age thirty-five should make use of IVF or ICSI. In IVF, the outer membrane of the egg (the zona pellucida) is an efficient barrier in preventing the penetration of sperm that have DNA damage. In ICSI, the best sperm can be selected and used. We have found that both of these methods help couples where the man is older to achieve a pregnancy more quickly and also reduce the risk of miscarriage.

Analyses of sperm samples from healthy men have found changes as men age. The numbers of sperm and their swimming ability may decline with age, and there may be a steady increase in sperm DNA fragmentation as men grow older. Above age forty there is also a decline in the amount of testosterone a man produces. Some studies have shown that men over the age of forty have more than five times the risk of having offspring with autism, twice the risk of having offspring with schizophrenia, and twice the risk of having a child with congenital abnormalities.

The cumulative effects of lifestyle choices such as alcohol, smoking, drug use, obesity, and chronic stress begin to take a toll. Other diseases that in-crease with age also affect testicular function, such as diabetes, hardening of the arteries, and cancer and its treatment. In fact, a teenager or a single man about to undergo cancer treatment should bank as much sperm as possible to help ensure his future fertility.

The biological clock does tick for men. But healthy habits, regular exer-cise, and a balanced diet can help even an older man to preserve his fertility. And in this age of assisted reproductive technologies, all it takes are a few healthy sperm that are still capable of fertilizing eggs.

In the Future

Sometimes researchers make tentative connections to male fertility that re-quire additional studies. Although more information is needed, cell phone use and certain chemicals in foods and in plastics may pose a risk to a man's fertility.

Cell Phones

The number of hours a man uses his cell phone each day may affect his sperm profile. In a small study, Cleveland Clinic researchers noted an as-sociation between cell phone use and sperm quality. The more hours men from an infertility clinic spent on their cell phones each day, the lower their sperm count and the greater their percentage of abnormal sperm. Men who used their cell phone for more than four hours a day had the lowest average sperm counts and the greatest percentage of abnormal sperm.

The effect of cell phones on sperm parameters may be due to the elec-tromagnetic radiation the devices emit or the heat they generate. While there is a strong association between cell phone use and decreased semen quality, this does not prove a direct cause-and-effect relationship. Further studies are necessary to identify the mechanism involved in the reduction of sperm quality due to cell phones. The Cleveland Clinic researchers are doing a follow-up study in a large group of men that also takes into account other lifestyle habits and occupational exposures that might affect sperm quality. We recommend that a man not keep a live cell phone in his front pants pocket.

Chemicals in Foods

Over the years, possible causes for sperm DNA fragmentation have been suggested, but the exact mechanism for the damage remains in question. A class of compounds known as advanced glycation or glycosalation end products (AGEs) may be part of the answer.

AGEs are thought to be major factors in aging and age-related chronic diseases. These compounds are formed as the result of the addition of sugar to protein, a process called glycation, in the absence of water. AGEs are formed when food is cooked in high heat and turns brown, such as brown cookies, brown bread crust, and browned meats. They also accumulate naturally in the body, and that's why diabetics have a high incidence of nerve, artery, and kidney damage—the high blood sugar levels in their bodies accelerate the chemical reactions that form AGEs.

The influence of AGEs may go beyond diabetes and its complications to contribute to DNA damage of sperm. Irish researchers are developing strategies to diminish the accumulation of AGEs and protect sperm. These strategies could involve disrupting a step in the formation of AGEs or increasing the body's protection against AGEs, possibly through the use of dietary supplements. More research will tell how much of a role AGEs play in sperm damage.

Chemicals in Plastics

Polycarbonate plastic, which is clear and nearly shatterproof, is used to make a variety of common products, including baby and water bottles, sports equipment, medical and dental devices, dental composite fillings and sealants, lenses, and household electronics. A chemical in these plastics, bisphenol A (BPA), has been known to leach from the plastic lining of canned foods, and, to a lesser degree, polycarbonate plastics that are cleaned with harsh detergents or used to contain acidic or high-temperature liquids.

Some studies now suggest that exposure to BPA, which has estrogen-like properties, may put men's reproductive health at risk. A small, preliminary Harvard University study found an association between higher levels of urinary BPA and poor semen quality in men whose female partners were seeking fertility treatment. The men with higher exposures to BPA had lower sperm motility and more abnormally shaped sperm compared with men with lower exposure to the chemical. Other studies have found BPA in more than 90 percent of urine samples from men.

The early studies should be viewed cautiously, since more research is needed to define fully the effects of BPA on male fertility and to understand its mechanisms. BPA may also be among the risk factors for female fertility, which are discussed in the following chapter.

Another ubiquitous group of chemicals, phthalates, is used as a plasticizer in PVC products (most plastic wraps, tubings, and consumer products) and has been associated with decreased fertility in male rats, and possibly humans. Uterine exposure to phthalates has been shown to result in undescended testicles and hypospadias in animals. These softening agents are suspected to have an effect on sperm count as well.

Take-Home Messages

- If you have borderline sperm quantity or quality this may add to your fertility risk.
- Certain medical conditions such as diabetes, an undescended testicle, or lupus can impair a man's fertility.
- Prescription medications for heart disease, ulcers, or depression may affect your fertility.
- An unhealthy lifestyle that includes smoking, heavy drinking, being overweight, or high stress, among other factors, may play a role in your infertility.
- Chemicals in the environment may contribute to infertility or worsen the effects of preexisting genetic or medical risk factors.
- If you are a man over forty, you may be at higher risk of having offspring with genetic defects.

Three

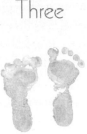

What Factors Determine
Her Fertility?
Risk Factors for Female Infertility

. . . .

Over the past decade, Elaine, a thirty-seven-year-old real estate agent, had kept herself very slim to look good for her upscale clientele. For many years, she had also subjected herself to a breathtaking array of fertility procedures, including taking powerful fertility drugs, being artificially inseminated with sperm from both her husband, Jack, and a donor, and enrolling in in vitro fertilization (IVF) programs twice. Her problem? She had irregular periods and was not able to produce very many eggs. Her husband's semen profile revealed a very low sperm count and very poor sperm motility.

Elaine visited Dr. Rosenwaks, who found that her hormone levels were quite low because of her low body-fat content. He suggested that she gain some weight, which she did over the next few months. A decision was made to proceed with another IVF attempt and to include intracytoplasmic sperm injection (ICSI) due to her husband's very sluggish sperm movement. Elaine underwent a stimulation cycle with follicle-stimulating hormone with a protocol specifically tailored for her. A moderate number of eggs were harvested and each egg was injected with a single sperm. Elaine successfully became the proud mother of her son, John, now one year old.

. . . .

A woman's fertility depends upon precise directions from the brain to start the flow of hormones that signal the development and release of an egg from the ovary. In the brain, the main hormones include gonadotropin-releasing hormone (GnRH), the hormone produced and released by the hypothalamus that controls the pituitary gland's production and release of two gonadotropins, follicle-stimulating hormone (FSH) and luteinizing hormone (LH). FSH stimulates the growth of the egg-carrying follicles and, along with LH, stimulates the ovaries to manufacture the sex hormones estrogen and progesterone. Another hormone found in the fluid of follicles, called inhibin A, inhibits FSH secretion. A handful of other regulatory and growth factors are also known to play a role in the regulation of a normal menstrual cycle. One of the other factors is called anti-Müllerian hormone (AMH), which may play a critical role in regulating follicle recruitment. AMH levels are very good markers of ovarian reserve, or how many eggs a woman still has, and can be measured at any time in the menstrual cycle.

A woman's body controls the normal monthly flow of reproductive hormones in a manner similar to a thermostat's control of heat in a house. When the house is cold, the thermostat sends a signal to the furnace to make heat. As the house warms, the thermostat senses the warmth and decreases its signal to the furnace. Similarly, at the beginning of the menstrual cycle, estrogen levels are low. In response to the low levels of estrogen, the pituitary gland secretes FSH. The FSH begins the process of follicular recruitment and stimulates the ovary to make estrogens.

The first half of the menstrual cycle, called the *follicular phase*, begins with pulses of GnRH, about one pulse every ninety minutes. A few days before mid-cycle (usually day 14 in a normal twenty-eight-day cycle), estrogen levels begin to increase. When the pituitary senses a high-enough level of estrogen for a long-enough period, it responds with a surge of gonadotropins. At this time GnRH pulses increase briefly and LH levels begin to rise, culminating in a surge of LH that triggers the release of the egg (ovulation) right at mid-cycle. Progesterone levels increase in the second half of the cycle, called the *luteal phase*, which signals the hypothalamus to slow down GnRH pulses gradually to every four to six hours.

The LH surge releases the egg from the follicle so that it can be picked up by one of the fallopian tubes. Only one of the many follicles (the fluid-filled sac containing the egg) stimulated each month matures fully and is called the dominant follicle. This follicle, at first the size of a pinhead, grows slowly over the first week. At the end of the second week, after the menstrual period, the follicle grows to the size of a quarter just before the egg is released at ovulation.

After the egg leaves the follicle, the round-shaped follicle collapses and becomes a corpus luteum (from the Latin "yellow body"). The cells in the corpus luteum secrete estrogen, progesterone, and inhibin A under control of LH. If a woman becomes pregnant, the corpus luteum continues to support the early pregnancy. If she does not become pregnant, the corpus luteum regresses, and levels of estrogen, progesterone, and inhibin A fall. The fall of these hormones allows levels of FSH to rise, the uterine lining is shed, and a new menstrual cycle begins.

Any number of factors can interfere with the normal hormonal production necessary to release the one high-quality egg and to maintain a suitable environment to nourish an implanted embryo. These include any systemic or general illnesses, stress, poor nutrition, excessive exercise, certain medications (especially anticancer drugs or radiation), recreational drugs, smoking, pesticides, as well as obesity and its opposite, being too thin.

The most important factor impacting a woman's ability to become pregnant is her age. Women in their thirties and forties are just not as fertile as those in their twenties. Aside from problems that interfere with hormone production and ovulation, achieving a pregnancy requires intact and healthy reproductive organs. Damage to the fallopian tubes, uterus, ovaries, or cervix from previous sexually transmitted diseases (STDs) or surgical procedures can all contribute to female infertility.

The Prime Factor: Age

Whatever the reasons, it is an undeniable fact that more women are delaying childbirth. As a result of this trend, an increasing number of older women now seek assisted reproductive technologies because they have been unable to conceive naturally. The decrease in fertility associated with advancing age may also contribute to the recent drop in U.S. birth rates.

Why does a woman's fertility decline with age? The answer lies in the number and quality of her eggs. At birth, a woman carries all of the eggs she will ever produce—1 million—in her lifetime. By puberty, the egg total has declined to about 300,000. The attrition accelerates, and by age thirty-seven or thirty-eight, her egg number has dropped to 25,000.

Chromosome damage in eggs becomes more common as a woman ages. These eggs may contain either too few or too many chromosomes. It appears that during the follicle maturation process, the factors that regulate chromosomal integrity are less efficient as women get older. This explains why women who are older have a higher incidence of miscarriage. Investigations of unfertilized eggs following IVF reveal that a woman's chromosomes degenerate at a significantly increased rate at older ages. Eggs from older women may show signs of DNA fragmentation and are more likely to contain deletions in mitochondrial DNA, that is, the DNA inherited exclusively from the mother, than eggs from younger women.

Chromosomal abnormalities are also the major cause of miscarriages among older women. Weill Cornell research shows that age has a dramatic effect on loss of pregnancy in IVF patients. An analysis of more than two thousand consecutive clinical IVF pregnancies, where an ultrasound scan showed a heartbeat at seven weeks, revealed that about 12 percent of women age thirty-four or younger lost their pregnancy. In contrast, more than twice as many women age forty and older lost their pregnancies. When we analyzed what had happened, we found that more than 90 percent of the older women's pregnancy losses were due to chromosomal abnormalities.

A woman's age also affects the number of embryos that successfully implant in the uterus. Our research shows that embryo implantation rates remain relatively constant until age thirty-four and then decline significantly thereafter. The implantation rate for embryos at day 3 is about 34 percent for a woman who is age thirty-four or younger, but falls to only 4 percent for a woman who is older than age forty-four.

In addition, an older woman's eggs have had more of a chance for exposure to drugs, chemicals, and X-rays. These environmental insults may also be responsible for abnormal chromosome division (segregation) in older women's eggs. This is why understanding the risk factors for infertility is so important: by minimizing your risk factors (no matter what age you begin to do so), you are maximizing your chances to conceive.

Lifestyle Factors

Just as with men, lifestyle factors may contribute to infertility in women. This includes any damage done by STDs, how many cigarettes a woman has smoked, how much or little she weighs, how she handles the effects of stress, and which of any substances she might abuse.

Sexually Transmitted Diseases

If left untreated, STDs can permanently scar the egg-transporting fallopian tubes. Most often STDs caused by chlamydia or gonorrhea travel up the vagina, through the cervix and uterus to infect the fallopian tubes, ovaries, and nearby structures. This condition, called pelvic inflammatory disease (PID), is often associated with fever, nausea, vomiting, severe lower abdominal pain, or pelvic tenderness.

About 1 million U.S. women develop PID each year. PID can occur at any age, but more than two thirds of cases are seen among sexually active women under age twenty-five.

It is estimated that from 10 percent to 15 percent of reproductive-age women have had an episode of PID. If a woman has had PID previously, she is more likely to develop another episode. About one quarter of women who have had PID will have another attack.

In the vast majority of cases, PID is caused by genital infections spread through having unprotected sex. In untreated cases, up to 17 percent of women with gonorrhea and 10 percent of women with chlamydia infections develop PID. Most women with PID harbor both gonorrhea and chlamydia infections. Various types of bacteria and other organisms, including genital mycoplasma and ureaplasma, have also been linked to PID.

PID refers mainly to an infection that involves the fallopian tubes. PID usually causes blocked fallopian tubes or scarring, called adhesions, surrounding the ovaries or fallopian tubes. The number and severity of PID episodes determines your risk of infertility. A woman has an 8 percent risk of infertility after the first PID episode, a 20 percent risk after the second episode, and a 40 percent risk after the third episode. What's more, up to 10 percent of women who have had PID who become pregnant will have an ectopic pregnancy, that is, a pregnancy located outside the uterus, usually in the fallopian tube.

The symptoms of PID infections may be silent, so the infections go undiagnosed and untreated, leaving behind scar tissue or damaging the delicate lining of the fallopian tubes. Most often, when a fertility evaluation finds a woman's fallopian tubes are closed, she was not aware that she had previously had a pelvic infection. Sometimes a man does not feel any symptoms either, and he may unwittingly pass the infection back and forth with his female partner.

Once a woman contracts an STD, her immune system reacts to the genital infection by producing antibodies against it. If the tiny organism that caused the infection attaches to a man's sperm, the woman's antibodies may attack both the sperm and the organism. A man's semen is recognized as "foreign" by a woman's immune system, but the fluid in the semen naturally inhibits her immune response. However, antisperm antibodies can arise when the genital infection overrides the protective power of the seminal fluid. These sperm-busting antibodies can also develop if a man's sperm has abnormal shape or structure or is already bound with antisperm antibodies. This in turn may spark an immune response from the woman's genital tract. Anal intercourse without a condom and ejaculation into a woman's rectum can also cause her to be immunized against her partner's sperm and develop antisperm antibodies.

If a woman's blood contains antisperm antibodies, they can bind to the sperm and inhibit fertilization. Although some studies have suggested that antisperm antibodies may be a cause of repeated miscarriages, this association is a tenuous one.

Cigarette Smoke

A strong body of evidence indicates that cigarette smoking negatively affects almost every system involved in the reproductive process. Cigarette smoking is harmful to a woman's ovaries, and the degree of harm depends upon the quantity and the amount of time a woman smokes. Chemically, nicotine has been shown to concentrate in the cervical mucus, and nicotine metabolites have been found in the fluid of follicles and have also been associated with delayed growth and development of follicles. Smoking appears to accelerate the onset of menopause by several years, which suggests that there may be a direct toxic effect of smoking on the follicles.

Components in cigarette smoke have been shown to interfere with the ability of cells in the ovary to make estrogen and to cause a woman's eggs to be more prone to genetic abnormalities. Smoking decreases levels of estrogen production and shortens the luteal phase of a woman's menstrual cycle. Smoking may also interfere with fallopian tube movement and egg transport from the ovary to the uterus. An association has been made between smoking and a risk of tubal pregnancies as well as an increase in miscarriages.

Heavy smoking reduces the chances for a successful IVF cycle. Nearly twice as many IVF attempts are necessary to achieve a conception in smokers as in nonsmokers. Women who smoke require higher doses of ovary-stimulating drugs, they have fewer eggs harvested, and their cycles are more likely to be canceled before getting to the egg retrieval stage. Studies also show that embryo implantation rates are lower in smokers than in nonsmokers.

Smoking appears to inhibit implantation of the embryo in the wall of the uterus by making it less receptive, possibly due to vascular problems or to a disruption in the stability of cells lining the uterus. A Portuguese study of women who received donated eggs found that heavy smokers (more than ten cigarettes a day) had a much lower chance of achieving a pregnancy than light smokers (less than ten cigarettes a day). None of the women's partners smoked and none of the egg donors were heavy smokers. The fact that the eggs were donated suggests that the problem was in the uterus, not the ovaries, of the egg recipients.

Secondhand smoke may also be harmful. Women who spend time with smokers may experience a greater difficulty in conceiving. University of Rochester researchers found that women exposed to secondhand smoke during both childhood *and* adulthood had a higher chance of suffering a miscarriage or stillbirth and a much higher chance of having struggled to conceive than women who had no exposure to secondhand smoke. Women who grew up with a smoking parent were more likely to have difficulty getting pregnant. The more hours of daily exposure to secondhand smoke, the worse these problems were. Other studies have also shown that exposure to secondhand smoke during pregnancy can increase the risk of miscarriage.

Exposure to secondhand smoke may be particularly problematic if a woman needs fertility treatments to get pregnant. Women who have underlying fertility problems may be particularly sensitive to the damaging effects of smoke. A preliminary study from McMaster University found that women smokers and women exposed to sidestream smoke had half the pregnancy rates per embryo transfer of nonsmokers. Sidestream smoke is the type of secondhand smoke given off by the end of a smoldering cigarette, as opposed to the smoke exhaled by a smoker.

Obesity

Too much weight can also affect a woman's fertility potential. A woman's chances of becoming pregnant steadily decrease the heavier she is. Obesity, defined as a body mass index (BMI) of 30 or higher, is known to be a risk factor for lack of ovulation. More than one quarter of women in the Western world are officially considered obese. According to Dutch researchers at the Erasmus University Medical Center in Rotterdam, the higher the BMI in obese women, the longer it takes a woman to conceive, even among obese women with normal ovulation who happen to be subfertile. It's also well established that a woman with a BMI of 30 or higher has a much higher risk of pregnancy complications. To calculate your BMI, multiply your weight in pounds by 703 and then divide the product by the square of your height in inches.

The relationship between BMI and pregnancy may involve the hormone leptin, which regulates appetite and energy expenditure and is secreted by fatty tissues. Leptin levels are increased in obese people, and there is evidence that leptin may influence the process of hormone production by the ovaries. Obese women may have disturbed hormone levels, which decreases their chances of successful fertilization and implantation.

Another factor that links obesity to infertility may be insulin excess and insulin resistance. These adverse effects of obesity are particularly prominent among women with polycystic ovary syndrome (PCOS). Insulin is the hormone that controls the change of sugar, starches, and other food into energy for the body to use or store. Many women with PCOS cannot process insulin properly. The excess insulin appears to increase production of androgens (male hormones), which are made in fat cells, the ovaries, and the adrenal glands. These higher-than-normal levels of androgens can lead to acne, excessive hair growth, weight gain, irregular menstrual periods, lack of ovulation, and infertility. About half of all women with PCOS are obese.

Researchers are beginning to understand the link between obesity and reduced fertility. British researchers recently showed that a gene implicated in the development of obesity is also associated with susceptibility to PCOS. This provides the first genetic connection between obesity and PCOS. In Australia, researchers have reported alterations in the fluid bathing the eggs before obese women ovulate. Abnormally high levels of fats and inflammatory substances in the fluid surrounding their eggs may impact the eggs' developmental potential.

Heavier women tend to need higher doses of drugs to stimulate their ovaries during assisted reproductive cycles. The live-birth rates from IVF become progressively lower as a woman's weight trends toward obesity. In younger women undergoing IVF treatments, BMI seems to have a significant negative impact on their fertility until they reach their mid-thirties. After age thirty-six, BMI has less of an impact on infertility as age takes over as the prime factor.

Stick-Thin Figures

On the other hand, a woman who emulates stick-thin celebrities also risks becoming infertile. More and more women are now shedding pounds as they mimic celebrities without realizing that dramatic weight loss could damage their prospects of becoming pregnant.

Superslim women who diet too much or exercise too much may have too little body fat to have a baby. A woman needs a certain amount of body fat to store estrogen and other hormones. A critical mass of body fat is necessary for normal hormone secretion, both in developing girls and in mature women during their reproductive years. If a woman's BMI drops below 19, she is likely to experience irregularities in her menstrual cycle. If she continues to lose more weight, she will stop ovulating completely. Also, a vegetarian very-low-calorie diet may induce menstrual cycle disorders.

In addition to reducing body fat, strenuous exercise may disrupt the normal fluctuation of hormones in the menstrual cycle and interfere with ovulation or menstruation. A stressful training schedule may also induce production of cortisol, a stress-related hormone put out by the adrenal glands.

Stress

Infertility itself can be stressful for a couple. You feel stressed because you want to become pregnant. Every month when you learn you're not pregnant, you become even more stressed. The increased stress could possibly further decrease your chance of conception. However, stress is difficult to quantify, and it is difficult to calculate the actual contribution of stress to infertility.

Changes in cortisol levels in the blood due to stress have been identified as risk factors for female infertility. Under chronic stress, a woman secretes more cortisol, and changes in cortisol levels from day to day have been shown to accompany mental stress. This reaction to stress may interrupt the production and regulation of hormones that are necessary for proper development of the ovarian follicle and ovulation.

The extra cortisol released due to stress is believed to interrupt the natural flow of hormones within a woman's body. The cortisol appears to reduce the output of GnRH from the hypothalamus. This can cause the pituitary to reduce its output of FSH and LH. This may weaken the signals necessary for follicle and egg development as well as ovulation. Research shows that cortisol can affect this hormone cascade at various stages of the menstrual cycle and thus disrupt a woman's ability to become pregnant.

Substance Abuse

Drugs that affect the central nervous system, including depressants such as alcohol and marijuana and stimulants such as caffeine, may impair fertility by modifying the output of hormones from the brain that control reproductive hormones.

Alcohol. Women who are heavy drinkers (two or more drinks per day) suffer from ovulation and menstrual disorders. In a prospective study of nearly 7,400 Swedish women, researchers at the Karolinska Institute in Stockholm, Sweden, found that the risk of infertility was significantly increased among women who consumed two alcoholic drinks per day and decreased among those women who had less than one drink per day.

Marijuana. Women who smoke marijuana have shorter menstrual cycles and shorter luteal phases. Chronic smokers may secrete small amounts of tetrahydrocannabinol, the active ingredient in marijuana, in their vaginal fluid, which can interact with and overstimulate sperm.

Caffeine. Even moderate amounts of caffeine—one to two cups a day—can lower a woman's chances of conceiving by 10 percent, and three cups a day may more than double that risk.

Medical Treatments

A number of medications or surgical procedures may compromise a woman's fertility.

Hormones, antibiotics, or antihypertensives can prevent an embryo from implanting in the uterus. If taken in the middle of the menstrual cycle, aspirin or ibuprofen (Advil, Motrin) taken to ease menstrual cramps may have an effect on the ovaries. When administered in high doses to animals, it has been shown to inhibit ovulation. Acetaminophen (Tylenol) can reduce production of estrogen and LH, impairing fertility. Antidepressants and painkillers may increase levels of the pituitary hormone prolactin and cause problems with ovulation.

Anticancer agents and radiation treatment may also compromise fertility. Some chemotherapy medicines, such as those in the alkylating agents group, can cause infertility. These types of chemotherapy medicines can be used to treat many different kinds of cancer, not just cancers that affect the reproductive organs. Chemotherapy can cause infertility by reducing the number of eggs in your ovaries or by causing early menopause. Radiation can cause pelvic adhesions and damage the chromosomes in your eggs. Many women who receive radiation therapy and chemotherapy for Hodgkin disease go into premature menopause because of damage to their eggs or follicles. Those exposed to both therapies suffer more damage than those who receive only one therapy.

Scar tissue commonly forms in women who have had surgery for a ruptured appendix, bowel repair, cesarean section, ectopic pregnancy, or the removal of an ovarian cyst. The scar tissue may interfere with normal function of the ovaries, fallopian tubes, and uterus. Treatments to burn or freeze abnormalities detected by a Pap smear can significantly reduce the amount and quality of cervical mucus and may interfere with sperm reaching the uterus and tubes. Multiple surgical procedures performed on the uterus, such as abortions, may also result in either weakening the cervix or leaving scar tissue in the uterus. Weakening the cervix could result in repeated late-pregnancy losses, while uterine scarring may affect embryo implantation and/or growth and result in miscarriages.

Environmental Impact

Exposure to the 87,000 chemicals in commercial use that are found in the air we breathe, the water we drink, and the food we eat may impair a woman's fertility.

Several epidemiological studies have shown that women exposed to pesticides may exhibit irregular menstrual cycles and reduced fertility rates, may require a longer time to become pregnant, and may have higher miscarriage rates as well as higher rates of stillbirth and children born with developmental defects. Women who work with pesticides, such as farm or greenhouse workers, may be less likely to conceive in any given month than women who have no occupational exposure to pesticides. But even women who have used pesticides in their homes have been found to be less likely to conceive each month compared to those who did not use pesticides.

Chemicals used to kill weeds (herbicides) and fungi on plants (fungicides) may contribute to female infertility by interfering with hormone signaling, disrupting embryo growth and implantation, or altering the chromosome integrity of the embryo.

Ethylene oxide, a chemical used to sterilize equipment in dental and medical offices, and solvents such as benzene, used to produce chemicals in volume, may lead to miscarriage among the female partners of those exposed to these chemicals.

There is also strong evidence that exposure to heavy metals, particularly lead, interferes with healthy reproductive function in women. Lead is used in batteries, ammunition, and metal products. The most common source of exposure in the United States is lead-based paint in older homes, lead-contaminated house dust and soil, and vinyl products.

Exposure to other heavy metals, including mercury, manganese, and cadmium, may also lead to reduced fertility. Mercury is used in thermometers, dental fillings, and batteries and accumulates in the food chain. The most common source of mercury exposure in the United States is contaminated seafood. Manganese is used in the production of batteries, in dietary supplements, and as an ingredient in some ceramics, pesticides, and fertilizers. Cadmium is used in industry and consumer products, mainly batteries, pigments, metal coatings, and plastics.

In the Future

Some of the effects of reproductive toxins are well known, while other, more subtle effects are still being discovered. Two highly ubiquitous chemicals, perfluorinated chemicals (PFCs) and BPA, may play havoc with hormones and the female reproductive system.

Perfluorinated Chemicals

PFCs are widely used in everyday items such as food packaging, pesticides, clothing, upholstery, carpets, and personal care products. They also are used in manufacturing processes, for instance, for industrial surfactants and emulsifiers. These chemicals persist in the environment and in the body for decades and may have a variety of toxic effects on the liver, immune system, and reproductive organs.

PFCs may interfere with hormones that are involved in reproduction. A preliminary study by University of California at Los Angeles (UCLA) researchers found that women who had higher levels of PFCs in their blood took longer to become pregnant than women with lower levels of the chemicals. The UCLA data showed that higher proportions of women with the highest levels of PFCs in their blood reported irregular menstrual periods compared with those with the lowest blood levels.

A man's sperm quality could also be affected by PFCs. This might contribute to the associations between PFC levels and time to pregnancy, since couples would tend to share the same lifestyles and have similar exposures. There's no data on PFC levels in men yet, though studies on sperm quality and PFCs certainly seem warranted.

It's possible that higher blood concentration of PFCs may be the result of another factor that affects fertility, such as obesity. Women who eat more packaged food and therefore consume more PFCs may be more likely to be obese, which might lower their fertility potential. Other studies need to replicate these findings to be able to list PFCs as risk factors for female infertility.

Bisphenol A

Originally created as a "synthetic estrogen" or man-made hormone, BPA was adopted by the chemical industry when it was discovered that it could make plastic light, clear, and shatterproof. Now it can be found in tin cans, plastic lunch boxes, plastic water bottles, baby bottles, mobile phones, DVDs, and thousands of other products.

BPA has been linked to male infertility (see Chapter 2) and has also been associated with PCOS, chromosome abnormalities in the egg, and miscarriage among women. University of California at San Francisco researchers found that BPA may have harmful effects on female reproduction. A pilot study suggests that women who did not become pregnant tended to have higher BPA concentrations. Their work shows that normal environmental concentrations of BPA interrupt the natural growth and maturation of cells lining the uterus (endometrium) and disrupt production of progesterone. If the endometrium does not develop normally, it may not allow proper coordination with embryo development, and implantation will not occur.

Estrogen-mimicking chemicals like BPA appear to have the potential to interfere with female fertility, but these preliminary small studies should be viewed with caution until this concept is examined further.

· · · · · · · ·

You and your partner can limit the damage caused by various fertility risk factors. We provide you with our guidelines on how to go about this in the next chapter.

Take-Home Messages

- If you minimize fertility risk factors, you maximize your chances of conceiving.
- Lifestyle factors such as STDs, cigarette smoking, weighing too much or too little, excessive stress, and substance abuse may contribute to infertility.
- Certain common medications, including antidepressants, antipsychotics, and narcotics, may compromise your fertility.
- Chemicals such as pesticides and heavy metals may impair your fertility.

Four

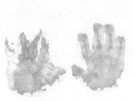

What a Couple Can Do
"Upgrading" Fertility in the Male and the Female

. . . .

"I've always been healthy in terms of eating a good diet, but I do need to lose some weight, and I'm working on it by exercising a little more. It just reconfirms my commitment to keep healthy. I don't drink, smoke, or do drugs," says Albert, a fifty-year-old banker who has just begun in vitro fertilization (IVF) treatments along with his wife, Sandra, a forty-year-old office manager. "I've changed my bathing habits to avoid too much heat. I only take short, not-too-hot showers and let the hot water hit my back, not my privates. I don't sleep with bundled blankets, and I've changed to boxers from briefs. I've also put away my bicycle until I get a wider seat so I don't crush my testicles. And Dr. Goldstein suggested I take a CoQ10 supplement every day, so I do."

Albert also pays attention to the stress-inducing events in his business life and adjusts his schedule to accommodate Sandra's IVF treatment cycles. "On days when I have to provide a sperm sample, I try hard to make that day not too crazy at work. I'll do paper work instead of high-stakes negotiations so I'm not so stressed," he says.

. . . .

Normal reproduction and fertility can be affected by seemingly simple lifestyle practices. Adopting healthy lifestyle habits to preserve your fertility may improve your chances of conceiving a child, while negative habits can contribute to your infertility. For example, many women cannot become pregnant because of inappropriate or unhealthy diets. Drastic weight-loss diets over time can affect the ability of a woman to ovulate and conceive. Recreational drug abuse can also affect fertility in both women and men.

The right choices in your daily life can make a difference in your probability of staying fertile. In fact, we believe that making changes to your lifestyle should be a first step if you are facing fertility problems.

Often, some negative lifestyle contributes to infertility in the couples we see. We regularly recommend that they live healthy lifestyles, and they usually see some improvement in their reproductive function after a few months. After changing to healthier lifestyles, many of them get pregnant on their own.

What a Couple Can Do

One of the simplest ways you can improve your chances of having a baby is to make sure you are timing sex for the most fertile time of the month. Ovulation predictor kits found in pharmacies can help you determine when you are ovulating. A basal body temperature chart may also help you identify your normal ovulation days and hormonal cycles.

When you do have sex, choose the right lubricants to combat vaginal dryness. Many couples use saliva, K-Y Jelly, Astroglide, Surgilube or other over-the-counter lubricants during sexual intercourse. But these lubricants, including saliva, can harm and may kill sperm, and they can create a barrier that interferes with the ability of sperm to travel through the cervix to the uterus.

Natural lubrication is best. We recommend the following lubricants: a small amount of baby oil, whole milk, or egg whites. Another option is Pre-Seed, a clinically proven, fertility-friendly moisturizer that mimics natural body secretions to relieve vaginal dryness. It provides an optimal environment for sperm and is delivered in a fluid that is mild on a woman's body. This lubricant is available for purchase online from http://www.preseed.com.

A Fertile Lifestyle

You can take control of your reproductive function by living a healthy lifestyle. That lifestyle can upgrade your fertility and increase your odds of having a baby. Here's what you can do to increase your chances of producing viable sperm and high-quality eggs.

Do Not Smoke

If you smoke cigarettes, you should quit as soon as possible. This will enhance your chances of having a baby, not to mention your general health and the health of your baby.

Smoking cigarettes is harmful to a woman's ovaries. The amount of harm depends upon the amount and how long a woman smokes. Smoking accelerates the loss of eggs and may advance menopause by several years.

Similarly, smoking cigarettes reduces the quality and quantity of sperm, can genetically damage sperm, and can also lead to impotence.

Stopping smoking really does make a difference. About three months after you quit, the levels of nicotine and other toxic chemicals in your blood and follicular fluid or semen will begin to drop, and in about one year the chemicals should be cleared from your body.

Limit Your Alcohol Intake

Drink no more than two ounces of alcohol twice per week. Large quantities of alcohol, particularly for men, may damage reproductive function. Men who are heavy drinkers risk having low testosterone levels, sperm abnormalities, and erectile dysfunction.

A woman should not drink while pregnant to avoid damage to her unborn baby. Heavy drinking can lead to major abnormalities in the baby and to fetal alcohol syndrome, which results in growth, mental, and physical problems for the baby.

Reduce Stress

If you feel as if you are under stress, consider meditation, yoga, massage therapy, or other similar relaxation techniques. Harvard researchers have found that practicing relaxation techniques regularly for six months can help infertile women become pregnant.

You may want to consider getting emotional or psychological support from a counselor. Many hospitals and community centers offer stress management classes. In these classes, you will learn techniques to deal with stressful situations and how to minimize stress in your daily life. The best fertility clinics also provide a psychologist or counselor to help you understand what may be stressing you out. If the stress has advanced to the stage that you feel depressed, it certainly is time to seek professional help.

Stress affects both men and women. It can interfere with the flow of hormones needed to produce sperm or eggs and can also decrease sexual function. Extreme stress may reduce sperm production and may impede ovulation.

Infertility and infertility treatments just add to the stresses of everyday life. As a couple, you need to work together to minimize any stress that you may be feeling. Try to support each other and talk about where the stress is coming from. Make time in your busy schedules to be together. Remember what brought you together as a couple and find relaxing activities to enjoy with each other. If need be, go to joint counseling sessions to work through your feelings.

Exercise Regularly and Moderately

Physical activity is good for your reproductive health as well as your overall health, but don't overdo it. A man who exercises to exhaustion may show a temporary change in hormone levels and a drop in sperm quantity and quality. We recommend that our male patients run less than fifty miles per week or bicycle less than one hundred miles per week to maintain optimum fertility.

For our female patients, it is generally recommended that they set moderate exercise limits. For example, training for or running a marathon can lead to hormonal defects in the menstrual cycle and may even disrupt menstruation and ovulation. The intensity of exercise, eating habits, body fat levels, and amount of stress a woman experiences may all contribute to menstrual problems. We evaluate each woman individually to make sure that her exercise activity is balanced by adequate caloric intake.

Watch Your Weight

You're most likely to produce large numbers of vital sperm and quality eggs if you maintain a healthy weight. Too much or too little body fat may disrupt production of reproductive hormones. This can reduce sperm counts and increase the percentage of abnormal sperm and can also interfere with ovulation. A woman needs to have a body mass index (BMI) of at least 20 for her to continue ovulating regularly. BMI can be calculated by multiplying your weight in pounds by 703 and then dividing the product by the square of your height in inches (multiply the inches by themselves).

If you are an obese woman or have polycystic ovary syndrome (PCOS), your body may be resistant to the hormone insulin, and insulin resistance has been linked to ovulation problems. If you lose weight, you can reduce this insulin resistance and may improve your chances of ovulating on your own.

Obese men tend to have low testosterone levels, high levels of estrogen, impaired fertility, and poor sexual quality of life. But if they lose weight, their sex hormone levels will likely improve along with their sex lives. University of Utah researchers compared a small group of very obese men with average BMI of more than 46 who had gastric bypass surgery to another small group of similar-sized men who did not have weight-loss surgery. Two years later, those who had surgery had lowered their BMI by an average of nearly 17 points and their estrogen levels fell significantly while their testosterone levels rose. And they all said that compared to their presurgery state, they were less likely to avoid sexual encounters, had less difficulty with sexual performance, and experienced greater sexual desire. The sex lives and hormone levels did not change significantly among the group of men who didn't have the weight-loss surgery.

You don't have to have weight-loss surgery to improve your hormone levels or sexual life. Similar, though less dramatic, results would likely occur if an overweight man lost weight through diet and exercise.

Eat a Healthy Diet
We recommend that a woman eat the freshest, healthiest food for three months before conception and for the nine months of pregnancy. The mainstays of the diet for you and your partner should be fresh fruits, leafy, green vegetables, nuts and seeds, beans and lentils, lean meat, oily fish, some dairy products, and eggs. Actually, it's like eating the way your grandparents ate—fresh foods untainted with chemicals.

A diet of too many processed foods and not enough fruits and vegetables does not provide the necessary fertility-promoting nutrients. Convenience foods are often low in vitamin B complex and essential minerals. Fresh foods are always more nutritious.

Proteins and oils from nuts, seeds, and oily fish (think of SMASH: salmon, *m*ackerel, *s*ardines, *h*erring) are precursors to hormones and enzymes. Eating a balanced diet, including adequate amounts of protein and fat, may aid fertility. A low-protein diet or a generally poor diet, on the other hand, may lead to poor hormone production and problems in ovulation.

The hormonal messages sent from the hypothalamus to the pituitary gland to the gonads (testicles in men, ovaries in women) are very sensitive to intake of the B vitamins. If these messages become weakened because of a lack of B vitamins, your fertility may suffer. Whole grains, such as oats, brown rice, and whole-wheat bread, contain an abundance of vitamin B.

Research suggests that antioxidant vitamins C and E are also important for fertility. Citrus fruits and also spinach are great sources of vitamin C and may help to enhance sperm quality by protecting against DNA damage. Avocado and whole grains provide vitamin E, which helps to improve the viability of sperm and to regulate both ovulation and the production of cervical mucus.

Other fertility-enhancing nutrients include selenium, zinc, essential fatty acids (EFAs), and folic acid. Selenium is a trace mineral that is important in sperm motility. It can be found in high quantities in Brazil nuts and in lesser amounts in tuna, codfish, beef, and turkey. Zinc is important in testosterone metabolism and in sperm production and motility. It is available in abundance in oysters and can also be found in baked beans, eggs, nuts, whole grains, and pumpkin seeds. Oily fish and flaxseed oil are great sources of omega-3 and omega-6 EFAs, which may help enhance sperm quality and motility. Leafy, green vegetables such as spinach are an excellent source of folic acid and may help to optimize sperm concentration and motility and facilitate healthy egg production.

Eating your fruits and vegetables can help ensure healthy, strong sperm. University of Rochester researchers have found that the more fresh produce a man eats, the more active his sperm are and the better they are able to fertilize an egg. For this study, forty-eight men with abnormal semen analyses and ten men with normal sperm counts answered questions about the food they typically ate. The clear-cut results showed that 83 percent of the infertile men ate fewer than five servings a day of fruits and vegetables compared to just 40 percent of the fertile men. Both groups took similar percentages of vitamin supplements, yet the infertile men had a significantly lower daily intake of vitamin C. Men in both groups who consumed the least amount of fruits and vegetables had the lowest sperm motility. These investigators suggest that men who are hoping to be fathers should eat a variety of fresh fruits and vegetables.

Take Vitamins

We believe that taking certain vitamins in moderate amounts may improve your fertility. The mechanism of action relates to the breakdown of oxygen as it passes through the cells in the body. This results in substances known as free radicals. Infertile men have a higher concentration of free radicals in their semen as compared to fertile men. Free radicals attack and destroy the membrane that surrounds sperm. Antioxidants fight against these bad effects, and vitamins are natural antioxidants.

A daily multivitamin can help provide zinc, selenium, and folic acid (vitamin B_9), three trace nutrients that are important for optimal sperm production and function. Men should take a multivitamin that contains no more than 20 milligrams (mg) of zinc and no more than 200 international units (IUs) of vitamin E. (High doses of zinc and vitamin E have been associated with small increases in the incidence of some cancers.)

We recommend that a man take the following each day: vitamin C (500 mg), vitamin E (200 IUs), selenium (200 mcg), folic acid (800 mcg), zinc (20 mg), and coenzyme Q10 (200 mg). Coenzyme Q10, or CoQ10, is an antioxidant that has been shown to increase sperm motility. One product currently available that contains all of these suggested supplements except CoQ10 is Conception XR Natural Conception Formula for men, available from http://www.fertilitysciences.com. It can be used with 200 milligrams of CoQ10 daily to fulfill the recommended vitamin requirements.

Two other supplements, L-arginine and L-carnitine, may be helpful for a man. L-arginine supplements, which are based on the amino acid arginine, may help improve fertility in men who have poor sperm motility. L-carnitine plays an important role in the metabolism of cells. Studies have found that consumption of carnitine may increase sperm motility, and some male infertility specialists suggest carnitine as a dietary supplement for infertile men with poor sperm motility.

Are dietary supplements safe? Many supplements, including vitamins, minerals, amino acids, and others, have not been proven to be effective in all infertile men or women. These supplements are generally safe, however, at the recommended dosages. We strongly suggest that you take the dietary supplements listed above, but if you have a fertility problem, you should not delay seeking other, more effective fertility treatment options. The above nutrients do not constitute the sole remedy for all fertility problems.

Do Not Abuse Substances

Stop using marijuana, cocaine, or other recreational drugs, which can adversely affect fertility, particularly if you have an underlying fertility problem. Marijuana stays in the testicles for two weeks, so even using it once every two weeks will have a negative effect. The good news is that most recreational drugs have only a temporary effect on the production of reproductive hormones. Once you stop using them, the harmful effects will likely be reversed in three to six months.

Do not use anabolic steroids. Their continual use can lead to low sperm counts and even complete sterility in men. In fact, testosterone has been successfully used as a contraceptive for men.

Reduce the Damage from Sexually Transmitted Diseases

The best way to protect yourself from potential damage from sexually transmitted diseases (STDs) is to have only one sexual partner and to use condoms during intercourse when you're not trying to become pregnant.

If a man feels symptoms of STDs—a burning sensation during urination and a puslike discharge from the penis or inflammation of the urethra—or if a woman feels fever, nausea, vomiting, and severe pain in the lower abdomen or pelvic tenderness, which are the signs of pelvic inflammatory disease, it's imperative that you visit a doctor for immediate treatment. Medical treatment can clear most genital infections and prevent further damage to delicate sperm-carrying or egg-bearing tubes. Your doctor may also suggest treatment if he finds white blood cells in the semen, which is another sign of a genital infection.

STDs can lead to antisperm antibodies that can prevent a sperm from fertilizing an egg. Testing for antisperm antibodies is indicated for a couple if:

- A semen analysis shows sperm that are clumped, not moving, or abnormally shaped. The presence of antisperm antibodies is the major cause of this problem. The female partner of a man with abnormal sperm or sperm bound with antibodies needs to be tested for antisperm antibodies as well.
- A semen analysis shows that the sperm count is too low or that no sperm are present.

In men with no sperm count (azoospermia), a positive blood test for antisperm antibodies helps your doctor make the definitive diagnosis of the blockage.

- Sperm recovered from the woman's cervix six to twelve hours after intercourse as part of a postcoital test are shaking or not moving. A poor result on a postcoital test is highly suggestive of antisperm antibodies. However, a normal postcoital test does not rule out the presence of antisperm antibodies.
- The cause of infertility is unexplained.
- The man has had a vasectomy reversal and his female partner has not become pregnant. Most men who have had a vasectomy develop antisperm antibodies. Once the vasectomy is reversed successfully, the antibody levels usually decrease gradually over a period of two years. If the antibodies persist, they can cause infertility.
- An IVF cycle is planned. Antibodies on the surface of a man's sperm or in a woman's blood that are used in the incubation medium can block fertilization. If antisperm antibodies are stuck to the sperm, IVF with intracytoplasmic sperm injection (ICSI) can overcome the problem (see Chapter 11).

If a man does have antisperm antibodies, low doses of steroids such as prednisone, which is commonly used to treat severe allergies, asthma, and autoimmune diseases such as lupus, can overcome them. These are not the bodybuilding steroids like testosterone that can hurt a man's fertility. Steroids such as prednisone should be used in low doses and for no longer than six months. High doses for longer periods of time can cause ulcers and even permanent damage to the hip joint (aseptic necrosis of the hip), necessitating a hip replacement. If the antisperm antibodies are due to a blockage, microsurgery to correct the blockage can reduce the antibodies.

Poor motility (swimming ability of sperm) may improve with a simple, inexpensive treatment with a nonsteroidal anti-inflammatory drug (NSAID) such as ibuprofen or naprosen. In addition to treating inflammatory conditions such as antisperm antibodies, NSAIDs may improve sperm production and quality by suppressing the synthesis of prostaglandins. Prostaglandins are chemicals found throughout the body that play a role in the contraction of smooth muscles. High concentrations of prostaglandins are found in the semen. Their presence in the semen may stimulate contractions of the female genital tract after ejaculation. By suppressing prostaglandins, NSAIDs may enhance sperm motility. However, chronic use of NSAIDs may have significant gastrointestinal side effects, including inflammation or irritation of the lining of the stomach (gastritis), nausea, and diarrhea.

Antisperm antibodies reduce but do not completely eliminate the possibility of achieving conception. Some couples can achieve a natural pregnancy even in the presence of antisperm antibodies. If a man's sperm are coated with antisperm antibodies, IVF with ICSI can overcome the problem.

Check Your Medications

If you take medications on an ongoing basis for some other medical condition, tell your primary care doctor that you and your partner are trying to have a baby, and ask for prescriptions that have the least potential damage to your fertility.

Chemotherapy drugs and radiation therapy can cause permanent infertility, but some chemotherapy drugs are less toxic than others. For women, alkylating agents such as cyclophosphamide (Cytoxan) lead to the highest incidence of ovarian failure. Platinum drugs (cisplatin, carboplatin, oxaliplatin) are mildly toxic. Other drugs, such as doxorubicin (Adriamycin), methotrexate, and vincristine (Oncovin), do not appear to have significant toxic effects on a woman's fertility.

The impact of chemotherapy on a man's reproductive health depends on the drug dose, duration of treatment, type of drugs used, and the severity of his cancer. Combination chemotherapy regimens tend to have much lower toxicity than chemotherapy with individual drugs because they use lower doses of each drug. This can reduce the damage to sperm cells and increase the possibility of restoring a man's fertility after treatment.

Surgical procedures can also help preserve a woman's fertility. If you need radiation to your pelvic area, you can have your ovaries surgically moved out of the field of radiation up into your abdomen and then put back in place. If you have early-stage cervical cancer, you can have your cervix surgically removed and still have a baby, although the baby will have to be delivered through a cesarean section. If you have stage I epithelial ovarian cancer, fertility-sparing surgery, with or without chemotherapy, can allow you to achieve a full-term delivery.

If you need to undergo cancer treatment, talk with your doctor about strategies to preserve your sperm and eggs. Sperm banking to store sperm for future use is essential for men about to undergo chemotherapy or radiation therapy. Many cancer patients have subnormal semen characteristics at the time of cancer diagnosis. It's recommended that more than one semen sample be preserved for future use. The more semen specimens frozen before chemotherapy or radiation treatments, the better off you are. Embryo freezing is the most successful option for women who want to preserve their reproductive function. This requires the woman to undergo ovarian stimulation and have a partner. In certain instances, a woman may choose to use donor sperm to fertilize her eggs to create embryos. Egg freezing is still considered experimental, although technology is improving daily. This is a reasonable option for a woman who does not have a male partner. If a woman's eggs or embryos cannot be frozen, she can choose to have part of her ovaries removed and the tissue frozen, with the hope of reimplanting the tissue at a later date, or she may have the immature eggs from the frozen ovarian tissue matured in the laboratory.

Limit Environmental Exposure

We suggest that you take some steps to limit your exposure to environmental toxins:

- Eat organic foods whenever possible. Organic foods, by definition, are grown with fewer pesticides.
- Try to eat a mostly plant-based diet. Eliminating most animal products from the diet helps to stabilize hormone levels and protects you from the harmful growth hormones found in beef.
- Install a filter in your home to ensure your water supply is free of bisphenol A (BPA), and do not drink out of plastic containers or cans, which are lined with BPA. This widely used estrogen-like chemical may have effects on both male and female fertility.
- Store food in glass, not plastic, containers and avoid microwaving food in plastic containers to limit further exposure to BPA.
- Avoid eating packaged foods. This will decrease your consumption of perfluorinated chemicals (PFCs). High levels of PFCs in the blood may lengthen the time it takes a woman to conceive.
- Watch out for workplace hazards. Certain workplace toxins might have an effect on sperm quantity and quality. These include heavy metals used in industrial processes, pesticides, and chemicals in solvents. Use protective clothing, proper ventilation, and face masks to reduce your risk of absorbing these toxins.

What a Man Can Do

The effects of aging on sperm can be slowed down by a healthy lifestyle, repair of large varicoceles, and possibly antioxidant vitamins. Men can improve their fertility potential with some simple lifestyle changes.

Avoid Excessive Heat

Keep your testicle temperature at normal body temperature as much as possible to maintain normal sperm production. That means avoiding saunas, hot tubs, and tight pants. Don't cross your legs when you sit, and get up to stretch your legs often during the day. Keep cool by wearing loose-fitting cotton underwear or boxer shorts. If you wear tight bicycle shorts, which may also raise your testicle temperature, try to limit your cycling to thirty minutes at a time. Do not sit with a laptop on your lap for extended periods of time. Do not keep an activated cell phone in your front pants pocket.

Get checked for varicoceles, the enlarged veins inside the scrotum that heat up the testicles. Varicoceles are the same as varicose veins in the legs and hemorrhoids in the rectal area. When they occur in the scrotum, they elevate testicular temperature.

Be Aware of Sexual Problems

Do not hesitate to ask for medical help if you have erectile problems. Impotence may be due to low testosterone levels but can also be an early sign of vascular disease or diabetes. A hormonal evaluation can help identify the cause. If you take sildenafil (Viagra) regularly, be aware that it may affect your sperm function and fertility.

Do Not Take Hair-Growth Medication

Put aside your vanity to increase your virility, and fertility. A small percentage of men who use finasteride (Propecia or the stronger version, Proscar) to regrow hair on their heads become impotent and have decreased semen volume. It's not worth the fertility risk to continue using it. Use topical minoxidil (Rogaine) instead.

What a Woman Can Do

Women also can limit fertility problems by making a few simple lifestyle changes.

Limit Caffeine Consumption

Drink only one or two cups of caffeinated beverages each day. Any more than that reduces your chances of conceiving. That includes coffee, tea (both black and green), sodas, and energy drinks. Be careful about hidden caffeine in dark chocolate, baking chocolate, and candy bars. Most painkillers also contain caffeine, as do certain cold medications, diet pills, and allergy medications.

Maintain Some Body Fat

Do not exercise excessively, diet extensively, or eat a very-low-calorie diet. These can all reduce a woman's body-fat level so far that she stops menstruating or ovulating.

In the Future

Some experimental research indicates that specific foods may help reduce the number of a man's sperm that have chromosome damage. On the other hand, other foods may lower his sperm count. Studies also show that a special diet may help women with ovulation problems.

Increased Folate Intake for Men

If a man gets enough folate in his diet, he may decrease his risks of producing sperm with too few or too many chromosomes, sperm that are more likely to lead to birth defects and miscarriages. The health benefits of folate for women have long been known, since too little folate in the diet may lead to birth defects such as spina bifida and miscarriages. University of California at Berkeley researchers examined the sperm from eighty-nine healthy men to look for different kinds of genetic abnormalities. They found that men who consumed the most folate had a 20 percent to 30 percent lower frequency of several types of sperm abnormalities compared with men who consumed less folate.

The researchers advise men who are thinking about becoming fathers to increase their folate intake, which can be done by eating more folate-rich foods, such as spinach, beans, chickpeas, and lentils, or taking a vitamin supplement. We already recommend that our male patients take 800 micrograms of folic acid, which is twice the recommended daily intake for women, to ensure a normal sperm count and motility.

The above study is the first to look at the effects of diet on chromosomal abnormalities in sperm. Before fathers-to-be start popping more folic acid supplements, we caution that this study found only a link, not a cause-and-effect relationship, between folate and chromosomal abnormalities. We can't yet say that increasing folate in your diet will lead to healthier sperm, but there is enough evidence to justify a larger clinical trial in men to examine the relationship between folate levels in their diet and chromosomal abnormalities in their sperm. This information could then help set dietary folate levels that may reduce the risk of miscarriage or birth defects linked to fathers.

Soy Foods and Lower Sperm Counts

Overweight or obese men who eat just a half serving of soy foods daily may have diminished sperm counts, according to Harvard researchers. Soy foods contain high amounts of isoflavones, compounds that mimic the effects of estrogen in the body. Animal studies have linked the high consumption of isoflavones with infertility in animals, but so far there has been little evidence of their effect in humans.

The researchers collected data on ninety-nine men who attended a fertility clinic for evaluation for subfertility. They asked the men about how much of fifteen soy-based foods they had eaten in the previous three months, including such foods as tofu, tempeh, and soy milk. Those men who consumed half a serving of soy foods each day—about the equivalent of one cup of soy milk or one serving of tofu or soy burgers every other day—had a sperm count of 65 million on average. That is about 40 percent less than the sperm counts of the men who did not eat soy foods.

Almost three quarters of the men with lower sperm counts were overweight or obese. Men with high levels of body fat produce more estrogen than slimmer men, and it might be that the extra estrogen from the soy interfered with hormonal signals and led to the lower sperm counts.

The sperm counts, even for the overweight and obese men, were still in the normal range, and the Harvard researchers consider the findings preliminary and inconclusive until they can firm up the results in a randomized trial. But if you are overweight, have abnormal semen parameters, and consume a lot of soy foods, it may be wise to cut back on the amount of soy you eat.

The Ovulation Diet

The same Harvard researchers have also come up with a diet plan designed around the idea that what you eat and drink can impact the reproductive system, in particular ovulation. It's based on research on more than 17,000 women in the famous Nurses' Health Study, which has tracked a population of women nurses for more than twenty years. The study found that women had a lower risk of infertility if they ate a diet filled with low-fat foods (except for some high-fat dairy, like ice cream), whole grains, and vegetables and took vitamin and mineral supplements.

The researchers suggest that ten simple lifestyle changes can boost fertility for women with ovulation-related infertility. But it's a huge leap to go from a statistical correlation to giving advice. While their observation is interesting—and we recommend a similar healthy diet and specific vitamins and minerals—their results do not prove that certain foods prevent infertility. They would have to take a group of women diagnosed with infertility and randomly put half on their diet and half on a regular diet and then compare conception rates. What's more, problems with ovulation account for only about one quarter of all female infertility. The diet won't help a couple with male fertility problems, which the researchers acknowledge, nor if the woman has blocked fallopian tubes or fibroids that impair the lining of her uterus.

．．．．．．．

If you and your partner are still having trouble having a baby, you might ask your family doctor, gynecologist, or urologist to do some basic tests of your fertility. If basic tests indicate a potential problem or if you've tried unprotected sex for at least six months at the optimal time without getting pregnant, then it's probably time to find a fertility specialist. You can find the right doctor with the information in the following chapter.

Take-Home Messages

- To optimize your chances of producing viable sperm and high-quality eggs, live a fertile lifestyle: don't smoke, limit your drinking, minimize stress, be physically active, maintain a healthy weight, eat lots of fresh fruits and leafy green vegetables, take fertility-enhancing vitamins, and avoid recreational drugs.
- Protect yourself from damage from sexually transmitted diseases.
- If you take prescription medications regularly or you need cancer therapy, talk with your doctor about strategies to preserve your sperm or eggs.
- Reduce your exposure to environmental hazards.
- If you are a man, avoid activities that raise the temperature of your testicles, ask your doctor for help with erectile problems, and don't take hair-growth pills.
- If you are a woman, don't drink more than two cups of caffeinated beverages a day and maintain a healthy balance of physical activity and food intake.

Five

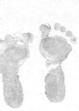

Who's on Your Team?
How to Find the Right Doctors

· · · · · · · · · ·

"When I was almost thirty-nine and about to be married, I told my ob-gyn I wanted to get pregnant quickly," says Andrea. "She suggested that I see a fertility specialist sooner rather than later." After trying for a few months naturally, with no success, Andrea and her husband, Gregory, age thirty-three, received a recommendation from her ob-gyn to see a fertility specialist, who suggested they try intrauterine insemination (IUI). Three IUI cycles failed, so the specialist suggested in vitro fertilization (IVF).

The first IVF cycle was canceled when Andrea's levels of follicle-stimulating hormone (FSH) became too high. "Before the second cycle, I started getting negative feedback from the doctor. She told me she had never seen someone my age with my FSH levels get pregnant," says Andrea. When the second IVF cycle ended in a miscarriage, "the doctor lost interest in us. It was difficult to speak to her. Whenever I called, she would never call back. She had a defeatist attitude, with no suggestions on how to tweak the ovulation drugs. Right then I decided I needed to see another doctor," she says.

A work friend told Andrea that her sister, who was about the same age and also had high FSH levels, had gone to Weill Cornell. Andrea and Gregory went to see a Weill Cornell physician. "He struck us as extremely thoughtful and highly scientific. He listened to our concerns, did not offer false hope, but was open and positive," Andrea says. And when I told him the other doctor had said she *had never seen someone my age with such high FSH levels have a baby, he took a deep breath and said, 'Well, I have.' "*

Andrea's first IVF cycle at Weill Cornell ended without an embryo transfer, but in her second cycle, using a special medium to co-culture her embryos, five eggs were retrieved, three were fertilized, and two embryos were transferred. Both embryos developed, and she gave birth to twin girls. "Having twins is exhausting and overwhelming at times, but I still can't believe I was able to have them," says Andrea.

. . . .

Two key factors in successful fertility treatments are educating yourselves and finding the right doctor. It's important to find a doctor who can come up with a treatment plan tailored to your needs and be sensitive enough to help you through what may be some rough times. Both partners should be on the same page when deciding whom you will choose to help you with such a huge life decision as having a baby.

Many couples suffering fertility problems start with the woman going to her obstetrician-gynecologist and leave the man behind. But it's important to find a fertility specialist who deals with both the man and the woman. In this chapter, we show you how to locate a fertility specialist, what to look for in a fertility clinic, and the hard questions you must ask the fertility specialist on such topics as credentials, experience, and insurance coverage.

Finding the Right Doctor

Anyone can put a shingle on the office door that says "fertility specialist"— even a doctor with no special training. Certain doctors have the basic knowledge to begin infertility treatments, while others have specialized training that allows them to treat more advanced problems.

Most women begin with their gynecologist, and men consult their primary care doctor. This is fine for a first consultation and maybe even for an initial infertility diagnosis or some preliminary treatment. If your insurance carrier covers fertility treatments, you may need a referral from your primary doctor before seeing a specialist.

Gynecologists provide specialized evaluation and treatment of women's diseases, including caring for pregnant women. To become board-certified,

a gynecologist must have at least four years of additional residency training and pass the oral and written examinations of the American Board of
Obstetrics and Gynecology (ABOG). Your gynecologist can perform some
basic tests, such as a pelvic exam, monitor baseline hormone levels, and help
you time sex around ovulation. Most gynecologists are also knowledgeable
in performing some early fertility tests, including a postcoital test, endometrial biopsy, and diagnostic laparoscopy.

Urologists treat disorders of the urinary tract in men and women and the
reproductive system of men. They perform the retrieval of sperm or other
surgeries, including vasectomy reversal and varicocele repair, to optimize a
man's reproductive health. Similar to a gynecologist, a urologist must complete one to two years of general surgical training and an additional three
to five years of urology residency training and must pass oral and written
examinations of the American Board of Urology.

Most fertility clinics don't pay enough attention to the role of urologists
in infertility evaluations and treatments. Male-factor infertility is mentioned
on less than two thirds of infertility clinic Web sites, according to a study by
University of Wisconsin researchers. Urologists who have training in male
infertility are rarely part of fertility clinic teams, and when male-factor infertility is mentioned on fertility clinic Web sites, the information presented
is either wrong or biased at least 12 percent of the time.

The Wisconsin researchers looked at data from the nearly four hundred
fertility clinics listed in the database of the American Society for Reproductive Medicine's (ASRM's) Society for Assisted Reproductive Technology
(SART), a subspecialty group that most IVF doctors join. They found that
350 of these clinics listed Web sites. Only two thirds of the academic clinics
and just over half of the private clinics mentioned that they treated male-
factor infertility. Twice as many academic clinics had a urologist on staff
(13%) as did the private clinics (6%), and the academic clinics (14%) were
more likely to have a link to a urologist's Web site than the private clinics
(4%). Surprisingly, less than one in five clinics even mentioned vasectomy
reversal.

Since infertility involves the male 50 percent of the time—40 percent
male factor alone, and another 10 percent a combination of male and female
factors—you need a urologist who knows how to handle the common and
uncommon issues that may come up.

If your doctors believe they have done everything they can, and you still haven't conceived, then ask for a referral to a specialist such as a reproductive endocrinologist or male reproductive urologist.

Reproductive endocrinologists are gynecologists with special expertise in the treatment of hormonal diseases of women and assisted reproductive technologies (ART) such as IVF or intracytoplasmic sperm injection (ICSI). A physician who is board-certified in reproductive endocrinology and infertility has done a fellowship that involves three additional years of specialized training after the doctor has completed obstetrics and gynecology residency training. The reproductive endocrinologist must pass both written and oral examinations and meet strict requirements for ongoing medical education and testing of a subspecialty division of the ABOG, including training in reproductive endocrinology and infertility.

Reproductive surgeons are either gynecologists or urologists with specialized training in fertility problems, including a familiarity with microsurgical reconstructive surgery. A gynecologist who becomes a reproductive surgeon is qualified to treat such issues as obstructed fallopian tubes, endometriosis, and structural abnormalities that require surgery. A urological surgeon has completed one to two years of specialized fellowship training in male reproductive medicine and surgery after completing urology residency training and knows how to repair blocked sperm-carrying tubes and varicoceles, retrieve sperm, and treat testicle disorders of an anatomical nature.

Other health care professionals in a fertility clinic—including embryologists, andrologists, reproductive nurses, genetic counselors, and psychologists—also care for patients.

Embryologists are in charge of the evaluation of sperm and egg quality, performing IVF laboratory procedures and the evaluation of the quality of embryos. They are usually not medical doctors (MDs) but are highly trained in advanced laboratory techniques and have earned advanced degrees in biology or biochemistry. Embryologists are also actively involved in the cryopreservation of sperm, eggs, and embryos.

Andrologists have specialized knowledge of male reproductive medicine and biology. They are usually basic or clinical scientists who are laboratory specialists and have earned an advanced degree in biochemistry, endrocrinology, or physiology. Their job in the fertility laboratory is to assess problems related to sperm production and function and to make sure the sperm gets together with the egg in ART procedures.

Reproductive nurses are specially trained nurses who actively manage a couple's fertility treatment. The reproductive nurse can provide answers to specific questions and serve as a liaison between you and the fertility doctors. You may be in close, if not daily, contact with the reproductive nurse during your IVF cycle. The nurse generally has a thorough knowledge of how the fertility clinic works and can provide you with additional care if you have special cultural, religious, or social needs.

At most fertility clinics, reproductive nurses teach you the correct method and technique for taking medication and how to administer injections of fertility drugs. The nurse will show you how to give yourself medications at home either intramuscularly (an injection into a muscle) or, as many patients prefer, subcutaneously (just under the skin). Most IVF medications available today can be administered by subcutaneous injection. In fact, most of the medications are so user-friendly that women often do not even need the assistance of their partners to give themselves daily medications.

Reproductive nurses are also quite helpful if you live in a town at a distance from the fertility clinic. After egg harvesting and embryo transfer, any blood tests for monitoring can be done in your hometown. The reproductive nurse can provide you with the necessary forms to have all testing done outside the fertility clinic and to arrange for results to be forwarded to your fertility doctors.

Genetic counselors have training in all areas of pregnancy-related genetics. Their role is to provide counseling if you are at risk for passing along a genetic disorder to your offspring. The genetic counselor works with your physician and focuses on your family's genetic disorders. The counselor also provides psychological counseling and support to help you adapt and adjust to the impact and implications of any genetic disorders in question.

Common indications for referral to a genetic counselor at a fertility clinic include two or more miscarriages; a history of stillbirth; the need for advice regarding prenatal diagnosis; a previous child with multiple birth defects, developmental delay, mental retardation, or autism; and a family history of a hereditary condition such as neurofibromatosis, cystic fibrosis, Marfan syndrome, sickle cell anemia, and thalassemia, to name a few.

You may also be referred to a genetic counselor if you have a positive genetic diagnostic or screening test that indicates you may be a carrier for a disorder. Some conditions are more prevalent in certain ethnic groups, and those groups would undergo screening to check on whether they carry the condition. Examples include screening for Tay-Sachs disease and Canavan disease among Ashkenazi Jews (those of Eastern-European descent), beta-thalassemia among those whose ancestors came from the Mediterranean, and sickle cell anemia among African Americans.

Certain chromosomal disorders are known to be associated with infertility. These disorders include men or women who have more or fewer than the normal forty-six chromosomes and those with deletions, or gaps, in their chromosomes. Examples include Klinefelter syndrome and microdeletion in the Y chromosome among men and Turner syndrome and specific deletions in the X chromosome among women.

In addition, a disorder in a single, specific gene may lead to either female or male infertility. This includes women with fragile X syndrome, who are at increased risk for developing ovarian failure, and those with Swyer syndrome, who have no functioning gonads (sex organs). In addition, this includes men with androgen resistance, who produce no sperm, and men with the cystic fibrosis gene mutation, who may have no vas deferens to transport sperm.

Psychologists are often needed to help couples handle the stress of undergoing fertility treatments. Most fertility clinics have a clinical psychologist or a social worker available for counseling. A psychologist can provide special support for your emotional needs. For example, a psychologist can help you discuss any burden your fertility treatment places on your relationship and how to deal with it. If the time comes to acknowledge that you may never have a biological child together, a psychologist can help you work through your feelings and act as a resource if you choose to use donor sperm, donor eggs, or adoption. For more on coping with infertility, see Chapter 17.

Going Straight to a Fertility Specialist

Once you and your partner have had basic workups that indicate there may be one or more fertility problems, some criteria suggest an immediate referral to a fertility specialist:

- A woman who is age thirty-seven or older. As a woman ages, her fertility decreases rapidly, so it is important to be more aggressive in treating a woman when she reaches age thirty-seven or above.
- A man who is over the age of forty-five. Male fertility drops with age, and genetic abnormalities in sperm increase significantly over the age of thirty-five. Paternal age over forty-five is also associated with a five times higher risk of fathering a child with autism, twice the risk of Down syndrome, and twice the risk of major congenital abnormalities.
- Blocked fallopian tubes.
- A previous tubal (ectopic) pregnancy.
- Moderate or severe endometriosis.
- A man with a history of undescended testicles, varicocele, hernia, or hydrocele surgery and treatment for cancer.
- Significant male-factor issues such as a sperm concentration below 10 million per milliliter, sperm motility of less than 40 percent, and poor sperm morphology (shape).
- A woman who has irregular or no menstrual periods.
- An abnormal ovarian reserve, characterized by high day 3 follicle-stimulating hormone level and low anti-Müllerian hormone levels.

Initial Consultation with a Fertility Specialist

Before you go to a fertility specialist, learn as much as you can about your condition by doing some homework. If you have a diagnosis of a fertility problem, make sure you know the potential treatment options available to you so you can discuss them with the fertility specialist and decide together what treatments to pursue. Be prepared for the possibility that some treatments will interfere with your daily routines; for example, some tests need to be scheduled on very specific days of a woman's cycle.

Most fertility clinics will provide you with a set of consent forms when you come in for your initial consultation. Many clinics have treatment and procedural consent forms that are center-specific and patient-specific. Generally, the doctors at the clinic will provide counseling and answer all of your questions before obtaining consent for any treatments. You should be able to raise any additional questions or concerns at any time with either your doctor or your assigned nurse.

Before your initial consultation with the doctor, make sure to send along all useful information, including all test results and your past doctors' reports. Use this first meeting to learn about the doctor's training and experience. Find out how long the doctor has been practicing and how many couples the doctor has helped; whether there is a nurse available or a call-in number to answer your questions; and what happens if you encounter a problem outside office hours. You should also find out whether you will see your doctor or one of his colleagues or associates during your treatments.

Most important is to ask what treatment options the doctor would recommend for you and why. If you are considering IVF, ask about the pregnancy success rate. Ask about the specific chance of achieving a live birth for someone in your age bracket and with your infertility diagnosis, and make sure you know whether the figures you are given are initial pregnancy rates, ongoing pregnancy rates, or live-birth rates. You want to know your chances of actually taking home a baby.

Your relationship with your doctor is important. Make a point of observing how much the doctor listens to you, answers your questions, and treats you with respect. One of the top complaints about fertility doctors is that they do not take the time to answer all of the questions their patients have. Trust your instincts about how the doctor's personality and approach mesh with yours. You should feel completely comfortable about working with the doctor.

First and foremost, a fertility specialist dealing with a female patient has to provide medical care at the right time of your cycle. Drug treatments need to be carefully monitored with blood tests and ultrasound examinations. That may include weekends and holidays, so the doctor or his or her team needs to be available every day of the week, particularly when you are ovulating. Depending on your natural cycle and the timing of ovarian stimulation, your egg retrieval day may fall on a weekend or holiday. Most large fertility clinics are fully staffed even on weekends and holidays. Some clinics may choose to time patient cycles to ensure smooth, consistent patient flow as well as adequate staffing.

Special Arrangements

If English is not your native tongue, translators may be available to help you understand all the details of your tests and treatments. If a specific translator is not available, you should bring in a family member or friend to translate for you during consultations or treatments. That family member or friend should also be available to interpret any daily instructions or messages left on an answering machine by your fertility doctor or reproductive nurse.

If you have an irregular work schedule, you can still maintain close communication with the fertility clinic. We generally encourage our patients to continue with their daily activities and work schedules. To maintain a close monitoring schedule during a treatment cycle, you may be asked to provide your doctor with your cell phone numbers, home and work numbers, and e-mail addresses. When an answering machine or voice mail is used to leave messages, our nursing staff asks the couple to leave an identifying greeting to ensure that the staff is leaving the instructions at the correct location.

Insurance and Cost Issues

Talk to your health insurance provider and find out if infertility tests or treatments are covered. Some insurance companies will cover infertility completely, some partially, and others will not cover any infertility tests or treatments.

How your doctor codes your diagnosis may affect whether insurance will cover it. Infertility is a symptom, not a disease. Whenever possible, your doctor should code for the cause, not use infertility as a diagnosis. Examples for women include endometriosis, blocked fallopian tubes, or polycystic ovary syndrome. Examples for men include varicocele, testicle atrophy, congenital absence of the ducts, or testicle pain.

If you have health insurance, try to select a fertility specialist in your health plan's network. Go through your insurance plan's directory of providers to find what fertility specialists in your area participate in the plan. You can check the provider directory either in booklet form or online.

Many fertility treatments are not covered by insurance, and you may have to pay out-of-pocket expenses. Request a copy of your health insurance contract from your employer or insurance provider. The contract will list what types of fertility treatments are covered and what procedures are excluded.

The degree of services covered depends on where you live and the type of insurance plan you have. As we write this, fourteen states currently have laws that require insurers either to cover or to offer to cover some form of infertility diagnosis and treatment. Those states are Arkansas, California, Connecticut, Hawaii, Illinois, Maryland, Massachusetts, Montana, New Jersey, New York, Ohio, Rhode Island, Texas, and West Virginia. However, the laws vary greatly about what is and what is not covered, and both the laws and offered coverage change frequently. The Web site of the American Society for Reproductive Medicine (ASRM) offers an up-to-date summary of what each state is mandated to offer or cover and whether IVF is included or excluded from coverage (http://www.asrm.org/Patients/insur.html).

For more information about the specific laws of your state, contact the state's insurance commissioner's office. To learn about pending insurance legislation in your state, contact your state representatives.

Make sure you know how much your tests and treatments will cost. Ask whether the fertility specialist offers any finance options or long-term payment plans. Ask for a copy of the fee schedule for IVF services, making sure that all procedures and fees are itemized.

Success Rates

Shopping for a fertility clinic is not like shopping for a car. One car dealer may throw in some extras, but the model you buy is basically the same as the one you would have bought from another dealer. Unfortunately, fertility clinics offer wide ranges of services with highly variable success rates. You want a fertility clinic that has high live-birth success rates as well as reasonable fees. But sometimes it's hard to pinpoint fertility success rates because many factors come into play, and clinics may provide data in ways that make comparisons difficult.

Two questions you want answered are: How many couples with our condition have you treated? And what is your success rate? If you need to use IVF, find out the fertility specialist's individual live-birth rate over the past year for all IVF procedures performed in women in your age group. As with the first two questions, get the live-birth rate for all cases of couples with the same fertility problems as yours.

In 1992, the federal government passed the Fertility Clinic Success Rate and Certification Act, which requires the Centers for Disease Control (CDC) to publish an annual report on ART (assisted reproductive technology) success rates. In general, ART procedures involve surgically removing eggs from a woman's ovaries, combining them with sperm in the laboratory, and returning them to the woman's body or donating them to another woman. This is IVF. They do not include treatments in which only sperm are handled (that is, intrauterine—or artificial—insemination) or procedures in which a woman takes medicine to stimulate egg production without the intention of having eggs retrieved.

Since 1995, the CDC has published the latest data provided by U.S. fertility clinics that use ART to treat infertility (see http://www.cdc.gov/ART/). This is a rich source of information about the factors that contribute to a successful ART treatment—the delivery of a live baby.

SART Data

Since 1985, more than half a million babies have been born in the United States as a result of reported ART procedures. IVF currently accounts for more than 99 percent of those ART procedures. The average live-delivery rate for IVF in 2007 was about 32 percent per egg retrieval—better than the 20 percent chance in any given month that a reproductively healthy couple has of achieving a pregnancy and carrying it to term. Since 2002, about one in every hundred babies born in the United States was conceived using IVF, and that trend continues today.

While all U.S. fertility clinics are required to report outcomes data to the CDC, this information is not individualized, is not verified, and may be a year or two behind the actual figures. The members of the ASRM's SART (Society for Assisted Reproductive Technology) subspecialty group voluntarily provide results from individual fertility clinics with the most up-to-date information available each year. For 2007, 358 clinics reported data to SART on 132,745 treatment cycles, 40,050 of which resulted in the birth of 53,050 babies.

On SART's Web site (http://www.sart.org), each SART member clinic has its own summary page detailing its procedures and success rates. The clinic summary pages allow you to customize your views of the data, sorting for diagnoses and treatment types, so that you can see the data that is most relevant to your own fertility experience.

On the Web site, you can click on the yellow box labeled "IVF Success Rate Reports" to search for SART member clinics in your area and view each clinic's individual data for various female age groups. Data is also available specifically for results using IVF with ICSI, which is used to overcome low sperm counts or poor sperm quality. Each clinic's report allows access to yearly data from 2003 through 2007 and details procedures the clinic offers, with corresponding success rates for women from under age thirty-five up to age forty-four. For example, the clinic summary report for Weill Cornell (https://www.sartcorsonline.com/rptCSR_PublicMultYear.aspx?Clinic PKID=1947, then locate Weill Medical College of Cornell University) shows that in 2007, using fresh embryos from nondonor eggs, 50.5 percent of transfers resulted in live births for women under age thirty-five.

You can use the Sart.org site's features to view clinic data organized according to the treatment types and diagnoses most relevant to you. Data from all reporting clinics is aggregated in the National Summary Report showing the big picture of ART in the United States. To track trends, previous years' reports can be accessed via a drop-down box.

However, it is critically important to know that the SART report does not identify the degree of complexity of patients treated in each clinic. For example, fertility clinics that deal with relatively less-complex infertility problems will have higher pregnancy success rates than clinics that treat patients who have not achieved pregnancy with treatment at other clinics. This makes comparisons between clinics difficult even for fertility specialists.

How to Find a Fertility Specialist

One of the best ways to find a fertility specialist is to ask discreetly among your friends or family members about doctors they have heard about. Frequently the same names will keep popping up. Ask for details about why your friends or family members liked a particular doctor or what they didn't like. The family physician, gynecologist, or urologist who saw you for early evaluations will also likely be able to make recommendations.

Other resources are readily available. Check with your local medical society for names of fertility specialists in your area. You can also find names of nearby specialists through the American Medical Association and the American College of Obstetricians and Gynecologists, which have searchable databases of physicians by name, city, or zip code. The *Directory of Medical Specialists*, which is available at most public libraries, also lists gynecologists and their specialty training.

Once you have the name of a fertility specialist, find out where and when he or she received medical training, in what field he or she is board-certified, and which hospital he or she is affiliated with. Many doctors have Web sites that will tell you this information, as well as how long the doctor has been treating infertility and whether he or she offers ART procedures such as IVF or donor sperm or donor egg programs.

The ASRM Specialty Societies offer search functions on their Web sites as well. You can find members of these subspecialty groups by checking out the following links:

Society for Male Reproduction and Urology
http://www.smru.org/forms/membersearch.html

Society for Reproductive Endocrinology and Infertility
http://www.socrei.org/SREImap.html

Society of Reproductive Surgeons
http://www.reprodsurgery.org/frsia.html

Society for Assisted Reproductive Technology
http://www.sart.org/find_frm.html

The American Urological Association also has a subspecialty society where you can find male fertility experts: the Society for the Study of Male Reproduction (http://www.ssmr.org).

For a fertility specialist who treats women, find out if and where the doctor completed a fellowship in reproductive endocrinology and if the doctor is board-certified in that subspecialty. For a fertility specialist who treats men, find out whether the doctor is board-certified in urology and whether the doctor completed a fellowship in male reproductive medicine and microsurgery. There is no urology subspecialty board certification in male infertility.

Is It Time for a Change?

Once you have started working with a fertility specialist, you may see some signs that this may not be the right doctor for you: your doctor suggests that you continue a course of treatment even though you've been through three or four cycles without success; your doctor dismisses your concerns; or you constantly have to remind your doctor about your treatment plan or to ask to have certain tests. If your doctor doesn't answer all of your questions or if you have to battle to book appointments for routine procedures, then it may be time to find another doctor.

· · · · · · · ·

Your fertility doctor will likely recommend that both partners undergo specific tests. For women, these include testing for whether you are ovulating (beyond basal body temperature), an evaluation of the cervix, uterus, and fallopian tubes, and occasionally laparoscopy to assess pelvic organs and rule out endometriosis. For men, your doctor may want to repeat the semen analysis, do special tests of sperm function and DNA quality, or perform a scrotal ultrasound. You will learn more about these cutting-edge tests and treatments in the next section of the book.

Take-Home Messages

- Know which conditions indicate that you should seek out a fertility specialist immediately.
- In your initial consultation, find out your treatment options and discuss them with the doctor.
- Know what fertility tests and treatments are covered by your insurance plan.
- Ask how many couples with your specific condition the fertility specialist has treated and how many took home a baby.
- Ask about the level of complexity and treatment technologies available at the clinic you choose.
- Ask your friends, family members, and doctors for recommendations on a fertility specialist. Search the Web for the specialist's medical training and board certification.

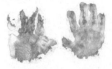

Part II

Cutting-Edge Tests and Treatments

Six

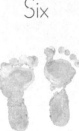

What Tests Should a Man Have?
A Male Fertility Evaluation

. . . .

Harold, a thirty-four-year-old copyeditor, and Lilly, a thirty-four-year-old doctor, had tried to get pregnant for six months, but to no avail. Dr. Goldstein's workup found nothing in Harold's fertility history that would have led to infertility, and his hormone levels were normal. However, during the physical exam, Dr. Goldstein found a large varicocele surrounding his left testicle. A semen analysis showed that Harold's sperm count and sperm motility were low, probably due to the varicocele.

"I had no idea I had the varicocele—or a low sperm count—but Dr. Goldstein said we would have a good chance of having a baby if I had varicocele surgery," says Harold. Under light general anesthesia, Harold had his varicocele repaired microsurgically. Six months later, his sperm count and motility had improved. "Dr. Goldstein showed us Harold's sperm under the microscope, and said, 'Look, they're swimming!' " recalls Lilly. "We were going on a trip to Europe, and he told us to start trying to have a baby." Sure enough, a few months later, Lilly became pregnant and the following year she gave birth naturally to their son, Lawrence.

. . . .

Infertility is defined as a couple's inability to achieve pregnancy following one year of appropriately timed and unprotected intercourse. As discussed above, the primary cause of infertility is a female factor in about 40 percent of these couples and it's a male factor in another 40 percent of them. A combination of male and female factors accounts for the remaining 20 percent. This suggests that a male factor contributes to infertility in 50 percent or more of couples.

Using conservative estimates, more than 2.5 million American men would potentially benefit from a fertility evaluation. The good news is that we can detect the cause of male infertility and then institute therapy in a majority of these men.

Historically, the approach to the infertile couple has started with an evaluation of the female, primarily because it is usually the female partner who initiates a workup by visiting her gynecologist. It makes more sense, however, to start with the male partner, since the initial fertility evaluation is much easier to do and is done quickly. The treatment of a specific "male problem" can be successful and at times less expensive than the assisted reproductive technologies (ART) treatments needed for "female problems" if the male problem is amenable to therapy. In addition, a small percentage of men who present with the symptom of infertility actually have a serious, underlying medical problem that may jeopardize their health or life if left untreated.

The man's fertility evaluation on the first visit includes a history, physical examination, semen analysis, and hormone tests. Even in this era of high-tech medicine, it has been Dr. Goldstein's experience that he can obtain an accurate impression in 90 percent of men in the initial visit. Almost always, he can identify the most common cause of male infertility—a varicocele, or enlarged veins in the scrotum—at that time. Varicoceles are found in about one third of men with primary infertility and up to three quarters of men with secondary infertility (trouble having a second child).

The Male Fertility Evaluation

The first step of the evaluation of the infertile male includes a thorough history, physical examination, microscopic examination of a semen specimen, and hormone tests. Some men may require further testing to confirm the initial diagnosis and help direct the course of their therapy.

Fertility History

Dr. Goldstein asks the man to fill out a detailed fertility questionnaire at home with his partner before coming in for his appointment. The history begins with an assessment of the couple's prior and current fertility status. One of the first things Dr. Goldstein discusses is the age of the partners. As noted above, a woman's age is an important factor in fertility success. After a woman reaches age thirty-five, the results of our in vitro fertilization (IVF) program show a steady, inexorable decline. We suggest a full fertility evaluation sooner rather than later when the female partner is over age thirty-five, either partner has had a history of infertility in a prior relationship, or either partner has risk factors that lead us to suspect a fertility problem exists—for example, the man previously had an undescended testicle, testicular cancer, or chemotherapy.

Dr. Goldstein's research, confirmed by others, shows that men with infertility and abnormal sperm counts have a twentyfold greater incidence of testicular cancer compared to the general population. If a man has testicular cancer, Dr. Goldstein recommends sperm banking before beginning treatment for this or any other cancer, in order to afford the man the opportunity to father children of his own in the future.

Next, Dr. Goldstein asks how long the couple has been trying to become pregnant using unprotected intercourse. For idiopathic infertility, that is, infertility of an unknown cause, your ultimate chance of success is often related to the duration of the infertility. The longer you have been unsuccessful in trying to get pregnant, the lower your chances.

The fertility history helps Dr. Goldstein establish whether the infertility is primary or secondary for each partner. If the infertility is secondary, he finds out the results of any prior pregnancies with the same or previous partners. He also notes the results of any previous infertility evaluations or treatments for either partner.

Sexual History

In about 5 percent of couples who see us for a fertility evaluation, the cause is sexual dysfunction. Dr. Goldstein takes a sexual history, asking whether semen is ejaculated into the vagina and whether the couple use lubricants, jellies, oils, or saliva, which may kill sperm. If the couple prefers to use lubrication, he recommends egg white or a small amount of mineral oil (baby oil). Because sperm can survive within cervical mucus for two to five days before ovulation, couples are advised to have intercourse before rather than after ovulation. Too-frequent intercourse or frequent masturbation may deplete a man's sperm reserves and can lead to infertility.

The sexual history also includes questions about the man's libido (sex drive), since poor libido can be associated with hormonal problems, increased prolactin, decreased testosterone, poor sperm production, and infertility.

Dr. Goldstein questions the male partner about the nature and volume of a typical ejaculate. A markedly diminished semen volume and clear, water-like fluid suggests absence of the seminal vesicle secretions. This may mean either that the man has an obstruction in an ejaculatory duct or that he was born without any vas deferens, which is known as congenital absence of the vas deferens (CAV). In a man who has normal orgasms with low or absent semen volume, Dr. Goldstein would suspect retrograde ejaculation (ejaculation backward into the bladder instead of forward through the urethra), and this would warrant an examination of a postejaculatory urine specimen for the presence of sperm.

Medical History

In the medical history, Dr. Goldstein looks for certain genetic conditions, surgical procedures, or infectious diseases that may lead to infertility.

An important risk factor for male infertility is one or two undescended testicles. This condition, called cryptorchidism (literally "hidden testicle"), is found in about 1 percent of newborn and one-year-old males. Fifty percent of men with a history of unilateral cryptorchidism and 90 percent of men with a history of bilateral cryptorchidism are subfertile. An infant or child who has had surgery to repair a hernia risks injury to the vas deferens. Adult men who become infected with the mumps virus can develop an acute inflammatory reaction in one or (more rarely) both of the testicles, which may result in severe sperm abnormalities.

Dr. Goldstein also ascertains whether the male partner went through puberty very early or very late. Precocious, or early, puberty suggests the possibility of an adrenal gland abnormality such as congenital adrenal hyperplasia, which can lead to excess testosterone. Very delayed or incomplete sexual development suggests hypogonadotropic hypogonadism, such as Kallmann syndrome, or testicular failure, such as Klinefelter syndrome.

Dr. Goldstein documents any medical conditions or illnesses as well as all of the medications a man is taking or has previously taken. Many prescription drugs can interfere with sperm development, most commonly cimetidine (Tagamet), sulfasalazine (Azulfidine), and nitrofurantoin (Macrobid). He also asks about cigarette smoking, alcohol use, and recreational drug abuse. The chemicals in cigarette smoke, alcohol, and drugs of abuse, including marijuana and cocaine, as well as anabolic steroids, can be directly toxic to the testicles and can affect sperm production.

He obtains a detailed occupational history to identify any exposure to toxic agents such as radiation, heavy metals, or pesticides. In addition, he finds out if the man has been exposed to testicle-damaging heat at work or at home.

A family history of fertility problems among parents and siblings may provide an important clue. For example, some women from the 1950s to the early 1960s took the synthetic estrogen diethylstilbestrol (DES) to prevent miscarriages. Their sons exposed to DES while the mothers were pregnant often developed abnormally small testicles, small penises, and missing ducts and may also have fertility problems due to low sperm counts, decreased sperm motility, and abnormally shaped sperm. Their daughters also suffered damage to their reproductive organs.

Physical Examination

After the history is complete, Dr. Goldstein conducts a physical examination. This is performed in a warm room with the scrotum relaxed by warming it with a heating pad. A relaxed scrotum allows him to more accurately examine the scrotal contents.

He has the man completely disrobe and stand with his arms outstretched This allows him to observe the man's entire body and his hair distribution in particular. Men who do not have fully developed secondary sexual characteristics (hair growth, muscle development, fully formed genitals) may not have much hair on their bodies or in the pubic area. They may also have disproportionately long limbs. This is due to a reduced production of the male hormones required for growth plates to close at the time of puberty. He sees this in men with hypogonadotropic hypogonadism or Klinefelter syndrome.

Next, he carefully examines the man from top to bottom (literally). He feels the thyroid gland in the neck, paying attention to size and looking for the presence of nodules. Both high and low levels of thyroid hormone production may lead to subfertility. High thyroid hormone levels can result in changes in testosterone levels, and low thyroid hormone levels have been associated with a decrease in sperm production.

He listens to the lungs and heart. Chronic bronchitis associated with congenital epididymal dysplasia is a sign of Young syndrome. Men with this syndrome have normal sperm, but the sperm don't appear in the semen due to an obstruction in the epididymis. A combination of chronic sinus infections, obstructive lung disease, and a rare inherited condition that causes the major internal organs to be reversed, that is, to mirror their normal positions, indicates Kartagener syndrome. This syndrome allows men to produce sperm, but the sperm don't move at all. A man who has enlarged breasts may have an estrogen-secreting cancer of the testicles, an adrenal tumor, or liver disease. A nipple discharge or tenderness may be due to prolactin secretions from a pituitary tumor.

He checks the abdomen by touching and tapping it. An enlarged liver suggests a liver dysfunction, which may be associated with infertility due to altered sex steroid metabolism.

Male Reproductive Anatomy

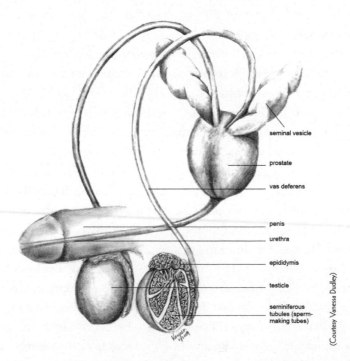

seminal vesicle

prostate

vas deferens

penis

urethra

epididymis

testicle

seminiferous tubules (sperm-making tubes)

(Courtesy Vanessa Dudley)

The penis and opening of the urethra are examined for genital warts, which may indicate scarring by the sexually transmitted human papilloma virus. He milks the urethra for any discharges, which may signal a sexually transmitted disease (STD) such as gonorrhea or chlamydia. He notes the location of the urethral opening. Men with severe hypospadias (an abnormal placement of the urethral opening) may not be able to deliver semen into the vagina.

The examination of the scrotum begins with the man lying down in a well-lit room. This allows Dr. Goldstein to assess the size and consistency of the testicles properly. He measures the testicles' size with a device called an orchidometer. This device has various-sized plastic orbs tied together like measuring spoons on a string. He simply matches each testicle to an orb on the orchidometer to size it. Dr. Goldstein jokingly tells his patients he's the only guy they'll ever meet who carries his balls in his pocket . . . and he has ten of them!

A normal testicle is about the same size and shape as a chicken's egg, and the consistency should be firm. In general, testicles that are normal in size and consistency usually have normal sperm production. In contrast, small, soft testicles indicate poor sperm formation. Small, hard testicles suggest a previous inflammation, atrophy from torsion (twisting), or Klinefelter syndrome.

Any firm, hard, or fixed lumps or nodules inside the testicles raise suspicion of malignancy. Smooth, firm nodules on the surface of the testicle usually represent a nonmalignant cyst. Mobile, small, hard bodies floating within the membrane covering the front and sides of the testicles and the epididymis are never malignant. They are calcifications, which are very common and are called scrotal pearls.

If the scrotum is abnormally enlarged, Dr. Goldstein turns the room lights off and examines the scrotum with a small, handheld light. This is called transillumination. This enables him to differentiate solid tumors from fluid-filled cysts or sacs of water around the testicle, called hydroceles. The epididymis, which runs along the center of the testicle from top to bottom, is normally soft and can barely be felt. An epididymis that is hard or has an irregular shape suggests an underlying disease. A full, firm, easily outlined epididymis suggests an obstruction. Shining a light through the epididymis helps locate any firm, smooth cysts in the epididymis, which are almost always located on the top of the epididymis and are never malignant.

After turning the lights back on, he feels each testicle for the vas deferens. The vas deferens should feel about the same width and consistency as a venetian blind cord. A little more than 1 percent of the men who come to see us have CAV. With a man's scrotum relaxed, Dr. Goldstein can almost always make the diagnosis of CAV simply by feeling the testicles.

Some men with CAV have kidney abnormalities or even lack a kidney. Dr. Goldstein always obtains a kidney ultrasound in all men with CAV. Most of these men also test positive for mutations in the gene responsible for cystic fibrosis (the *CFTR* gene), even if they do not have any of the digestive or lung symptoms that usually accompany this disease. He tests both partners for *CFTR* gene mutations and refers the couple for genetic counseling. All men who have full-blown cystic fibrosis have CAV on both sides.

Varicoceles

In a warm room with the man standing and the scrotum warmed with a heating pad, Dr. Goldstein can readily see large varicoceles through the skin of a relaxed scrotum. They look like a bag of worms above or alongside the testicles. Varicoceles are enlarged or dilated veins in the spermatic cord within the scrotum, similar to varicose veins in the leg and hemorrhoids in the rectal area. Blood pools in the enlarged veins and raises the temperature in the testicles. It's this rise in temperature that is believed to inhibit sperm production and affect a man's fertility. Typically, varicoceles are found on the left side, and in the 50 percent of men who have them on both sides, the left one is larger.

Varicocele

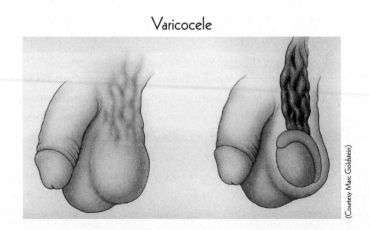

(Courtesy Marc Goldstein)

Smaller varicoceles take a little work on the man's part to diagnose. He must perform what's called the Valsalva maneuver. Dr. Goldstein has the man bear down as if he was having a difficult bowel movement or like a bodybuilder trying to make his muscles bulge. The squeezing makes the veins in his scrotum bulge out more to make it easier to detect smaller varicoceles.

If he detects a varicocele of any size, Dr. Goldstein has the man lie down on his back. A varicocele should completely collapse when he is flat on his back. A large varicocele that does not collapse in this position leads Dr. Goldstein to suspect an abdominal tumor, and he will send the man for an abdominal ultrasound scan. An ultrasound scan of the scrotum also helps in the evaluation of a questionable varicocele in an obese man or a man with a small, tight scrotum and is the best test for testicular cancer.

Size matters when it comes to varicoceles. Dr. Goldstein's data clearly show that men with large varicoceles have lower sperm counts but sustain a greater improvement in semen quality following varicocele surgery than men with small or subclinical varicoceles. His studies also show that varicoceles raise the temperature inside the testicles, and repairing these varicoceles causes the temperature to drop.

Dr. Goldstein ends the physical examination with a rectal examination. He notes the size and consistency of the prostate, looking for any masses, cysts, irregularities, tenderness, and whether he can feel the seminal vesicles. He also tests the man's stool for blood as a screen for colon cancer.

Semen Analysis

A semen sample should be collected in a quiet, private, comfortable room. The semen specimen is obtained by masturbation into a sterile wide-mouthed container. The doctor asks the man to abstain from sex for two to five days beforehand to optimize the sample. Two to three samples separated by at least one month are collected in order to get the most meaningful results. If the man has been ill with a fever or has been exposed to any agents that are toxic to sperm—for example, chemicals, medicines, or recreational drugs—he waits at least three months before repeating the semen analysis.

Normal semen looks like a clotted gel and usually liquefies within ten to twenty minutes of ejaculation. The normal ejaculate volume is between 2 and 6 milliliters, or about one half to one teaspoon. About two thirds of the volume comes from the seminal vesicles, which provide the protein that causes the ejaculate to coagulate. Another one third of the volume derives from the prostate, which provides the enzymes that liquefy the ejaculate. Only about 2 percent of the semen volume is contributed by the vas deferens, but that is where all the sperm comes from. That is why, after a vasectomy or a blockage of the epididymis or vas deferens from hernia or hydrocele surgery, there is no noticeable change in the amount, appearance, or smell of a man's semen.

If a man's semen doesn't look like a clotted, whitish gel, but has a low volume and is clear and thin like water, his seminal vesicles may be malfunctioning or even absent. If the semen does not turn into a liquid, he may have a prostate abnormality.

If a man has a zero sperm count coupled with low ejaculate volume and nonclotting, watery fluid with no fructose (which is supplied by the seminal vesicles), it's likely he has an obstruction or absence of the ejaculatory ducts. If Dr. Goldstein can feel the vas deferens, then an ultrasound exam can confirm this obstruction. Low fructose in the semen may also suggest an inflammation of the seminal vesicles or a testosterone deficiency. A complete lack of fructose suggests he has either no seminal vesicles or a complete obstruction of the ejaculatory ducts.

Men who have low sperm counts or low sperm motility with a low semen volume may have a partial ejaculatory duct obstruction or they may have retrograde ejaculation, in which semen is ejaculated backward into the bladder. To test for retrograde ejaculation, Dr. Goldstein has the man empty his bladder prior to ejaculation and then again in a separate container following ejaculation. If he finds lots of sperm in the voided sample, the man has retrograde ejaculation, which is commonly seen in diabetics as well as in men who have had prostate surgery or other surgical procedures near the bladder.

Sperm Quality

The gold standard for determining the quality of a sperm sample is to look at the sperm through a microscope to evaluate sperm concentration (the total number of sperm per milliliter), motility (the percentage of actively moving sperm), progression (how fast they are moving), and morphology (sperm size and shape).

A normal sperm count of more than 20 million sperm per milliliter of fluid is the most reliable predictor of fertility in a semen analysis. Less than 20 million sperm per milliliter is considered a low sperm count, which may be due to a variety of factors, including abnormal sperm production, hormone deficiency, varicocele, medications, childhood conditions such as an undescended testicle, or environmental factors such as excessive heat. But sperm quantity does not necessarily equal sperm quality. Many men with low sperm counts have good-quality sperm and with proper treatment can father children.

One measure of sperm quality is progressive sperm motility, or how strong the sperm swim. Only sperm with good tail movement can swim their way through the woman's reproductive tract and reach the egg. For normal sperm motility, at least 50 percent of a man's sperm must have good or excellent forward progression. If a high percentage of viable sperm in a sample have low motility, Dr. Goldstein suspects partial blockage and will order an antisperm antibody test. If semen volume is low, he orders a transrectal ultrasound to look for ejaculatory duct blockage near the prostate. Prolonged periods of abstinence can also lower a man's motility.

Another important measure of sperm quality is morphology, or shape. Normal sperm have a smooth, oval head with no defects in the neck, midpiece, or tail. Sperm with large, round heads may lack the acrosomal cap, the packet of enzymes that allow sperm to penetrate and fertilize the egg. Sperm may have many different head defects, such as pinheads or tapered heads. A consistent defect, such as all sperm with pinheads, indicates a genetic problem. Trauma, exposure to heat, and a varicocele can all affect sperm morphology.

The proper interpretation of sperm morphology requires an understanding of the scoring system and criteria used by the testing laboratory. Some laboratories use strict criteria (called the Kruger criteria) to assess sperm morphology. You need to know if your laboratory used standard criteria or stricter ones, especially if you are getting a second opinion or sharing those lab results with another doctor. In broad terms, profound abnormalities in sperm morphology are associated with poor fertilizing ability when strict criteria are used. Men with fewer than 4 percent perfectly shaped sperm usually cannot fertilize their partner's eggs without IVF with intracytoplasmic sperm injection (ICSI).

If the semen analysis finds 1 million or more white blood cells, this could mean infection or inflammation. Dr. Goldstein then checks for a genital tract infection by doing a semen culture. After the man washes his hands and penis with an antiseptic solution, he ejaculates into a sterile cup. The pH of the semen, which determines its acidity, can also be used to detect an infection. A man whose pH is high (more than 8.1) may also have an infection. A low pH (less than 7.0; very acidic semen) associated with a low volume and waterlike, clear semen suggests absence of the vas deferens or ejaculatory duct obstruction.

Semen Analysis Normal Ranges (WHO Criteria, 1999)

Semen Characteristics	
Volume	2.0 ml or more
pH	7.2 or greater
Sperm concentration	20 million or more per ml
Total sperm count	More than 40 million per ejaculate
Motility (within 60 minutes of ejaculation)	More than 50% motile
Progression at room temperature	3–4 (on a scale of 0–4)
Morphology	At least 30% normal sperm (at least 14% strict or Kruger). Greater than 4% by very strict criteria to be eligible for basic IVF.
Vitality	At least 75% live sperm
White blood cells	Less than 1 million

Because we can now achieve a pregnancy with only one sperm, any semen sample that appears to have no sperm is centrifuged and examined carefully for sperm. Even the presence of only a single sperm is a good prognostic sign since it means there are more sperm in the testicle or ducts, and a pregnancy is definitely possible using IVF with ICSI.

Semen samples that show sperm clumping (agglutination) of one sperm head to another or one tail to another usually signal the presence of an infection or antisperm antibodies. When present, semen cultures should be obtained to look for bacteria such as enterococcus, *E. coli*, and chlamydia, as well as mycoplasma, which may affect fertility. Reliable cultures require that the man makes sure to wash his hands, penis, and scrotum with an antibacterial scrub before producing a semen sample for culture to avoid contamination with the normal bacteria on the skin.

If there are no signs of infection, then Dr. Goldstein orders antisperm antibody testing. Men at high risk of developing antisperm antibodies include those who have had testicle torsion, inflammation of the epididymis or testicles, a partial obstruction of sperm-carrying tubes, and large varicoceles.

Two valid antisperm antibody tests—the immunobead assay and the mixed antiglobulin reaction test—measure the binding of antibodies to the surface of living sperm. Both tests can detect antibodies on the sperm, in the blood, and in cervical mucus. They cost from $50 to $150 per sample. In both tests, the greater the percentage of sperm bound with antibodies or the greater the number of sperm that acquire antibodies following incubation with blood or cervical mucus, the lower the probability of fertility without some form of intervention. The female partners of men with sperm bound with antibodies need to be tested for antisperm antibodies as well.

High levels of antibodies are most often seen when a man has an obstruction in sperm-carrying ducts. If a man has a zero sperm count and antisperm antibodies in his blood, then the outflow of sperm is likely blocked. The good news is that a positive antisperm antibody test means the man has to be making sperm, but they can't get out. He needs further evaluation that may lead to microsurgery to open up the blockage in the reproductive tract.

If a man has been taking selective serotonin reuptake inhibitors (SSRIs) to treat depression for a long time, he is over age forty-five, has had cancer treatments, or his wife has had recurrent miscarriages, Dr. Goldstein may order a sperm chromatin structure assay (SCSA). This new diagnostic tool can detect sperm samples that have a high degree of DNA fragmentation (small breaks in the sperm chromosomes). If 30 percent or more of your sperm are highly fragmented, then your partner may have more trouble carrying a pregnancy to term. Abnormal sperm DNA fragmentation is the only male factor identified with an impaired pregnancy rate using IVF. It's unclear whether this has an impact on ICSI outcome.

Evaluation of Hormone Levels

The next step in the fertility evaluation is to draw some blood to measure hormone levels. Our basic evaluation of hormones includes measurement of blood levels of testosterone, follicle-stimulating hormone (FSH), and luteinizing hormone (LH). These two pituitary hormones get transported through the bloodstream to the testicles and stimulate the production of sperm and testosterone.

Testosterone is necessary for the development and maintenance of secondary sexual characteristics, libido, erections, muscle strength, and energy levels. It also stimulates the prostate and seminal vesicles to make their secretions. Along with FSH stimulation, testosterone helps initiate and maintain sperm formation.

Testosterone exists in the blood in two forms—bound and free. About 98 percent of testosterone is bound to either of the proteins albumin or sex hormone–binding globulin (SHBG). The remaining 2 percent is free or biologically active. In most cases, free and total testosterone levels correlate with each other. But some conditions show increases or decreases in SHBG, leading to a discrepancy between free and total testosterone levels. Men with high thyroid hormone levels and those who use antiepilepsy medications have an increase in SHBG. Their total testosterone levels are elevated without an increase in biologically active or free testosterone. The opposite occurs in obese men, in which SHBG is decreased. Their total testosterone levels are low, but the free testosterone levels are normal.

Normal FSH levels in the blood can be helpful in determining whether a man's low sperm count is due to lack of sperm production or an obstruction in the reproductive tract. High blood levels of FSH mean impaired sperm production. When the testicles have enough FSH, the Sertoli cells in the testicles send the hormone inhibin to the pituitary gland as a signal to turn off FSH secretion. An FSH level greater than two to three times normal suggests a severe impairment in the tubules within the testicles that help create sperm.

Men with low levels of FSH, LH, and testosterone typically have hypogonadotropic hypogonadism. If the sense of smell is absent, this form of hypogonadotropic hypogonadism is called Kallmann syndrome. This disorder is usually congenital and first comes to light when the boy fails to go through puberty. It can also occur in adults who develop a benign pituitary tumor called a prolactinoma, and is associated with decreased libido and high blood levels of the pituitary hormone prolactin. High blood levels of prolactin suppress LH and FSH production, which in turn suppresses testosterone and sperm production. Some common medications, such as phenothiazines, imipramine, methyldopa, and reserpine, will also raise prolactin levels, as will excessive stress. So if prolactin levels are mildly high, Dr. Goldstein repeats the blood test. If prolactin levels are very high, he sends the man for magnetic resonance imaging (MRI) of the brain to look for a pituitary or other tumors. Rarely, this condition may be caused by a pituitary tumor.

If a man's testosterone levels are low, he also obtains an estradiol level. An elevated estradiol level may disturb the balance of testosterone and estradiol in a man's blood and may contribute to infertility. The ratio of testosterone to estradiol should be ten to one. A lower ratio may need to be corrected through therapy with an aromatase inhibitor, such as testolactone or anastrozole.

Normal Values of Male Hormones

Testosterone, total	300–1,100 ng/dl
Testosterone, free	50–210 pg/ml
Prolactin	0.1–15.2 ng/ml
LH (< 50 years)	0.5 10 mIU/ml
FSH	0.8–9 mIU/ml
Estradiol	< 60 pg/ml

< = less than, ng – nanograms, dl = deciliter, ml = milliliter,
mIU = milli–international units, pg = picograms

Values from the Endocrinology Laboratory at New York Hospital.
Normal values may vary in other laboratories.

Genetic Tests

Genetic testing is necessary for all men with zero sperm count or sperm concentrations of less than 5 million per milliliter. The first of two blood tests that are needed is a chromosome analysis, also called a karyotype, to see if the man has the normal forty-six chromosomes, including one X and one Y. The most common genetic abnormality in men with a zero sperm count is Klinefelter syndrome, in which the man has forty-seven chromosomes (47 XXY). This syndrome occurs in one in every six hundred newborn males. The next most common abnormality is a missing piece of the man's Y chromosome, called a micro Y deletion. This is diagnosed by the second of the two blood tests. Here at Weill Cornell, we have been able successfully to find sperm in the testicles and achieve pregnancies using IVF with ICSI in more than half of the men who have these genetic abnormalities.

Men who are missing all or part of the vas deferens need to be tested for mutations of the cystic fibrosis gene. If they are positive, their wives need to be tested as well. Those men almost always have normal sperm production, but the sperm can't get out. We are now able to help almost all of these men father children by microsurgically aspirating (sucking out) sperm from the little bit of ducts they have and using it for IVF with ICSI.

Testicular Biopsy

If a man has a zero sperm count, a negative antisperm antibody test, a negative test for Klinefelter syndrome, no micro Y deletions, normal-sized testicles, and normal blood levels of FSH, and Dr. Goldstein can feel (palpate) the vas deferens on the physical exam, then the man needs a testicular biopsy. This test will tell whether his zero sperm count is due to an obstruction in the sperm-carrying tubes or a lack of sperm production (nonobstructive azoospermia, or NOA).

A variety of conditions can lead to NOA, which is one of the most challenging types of male factor infertility to manage. Along with Klinefelter syndrome, other causes of NOA are cryptorchidism, low levels of LH and FSH (hypogonadotropic hypogonadism), high levels of estrogen and prolactin, thyroid abnormalities, previous testicular torsion, or a huge varicocele. What's more, environmental hazards, such as radiation and heat injury, radiation therapy or chemotherapy, infections or inflammations, and drug use may also lead to NOA.

To perform the testicular biopsy, Dr. Goldstein removes a tiny piece of tissue from each testicle and examines the tissue under a microscope. If he sees many sperm, then the man has an obstruction in the tubes of his reproductive tract. Careful microscopic reconstructive surgery can usually repair these blockages. If there appears to be no sperm production, then the man may have arrested sperm maturation or Sertoli-cell-only syndrome. Men with this syndrome, which is found in 13 percent of men with zero sperm counts, usually have small or soft testicles, well-developed secondary sexual characteristics, elevated FSH levels, normal or slightly elevated LH levels, and normal or slightly decreased testosterone levels. They lack the cells that produce sperm. At Weill Cornell, rare sperm can be retrieved from the testicles in more than one third of these men, and these sperm can be used for IVF with ICSI.

The testicle biopsy is a simple outpatient procedure that is usually done under general anesthesia. Dr. Goldstein uses an operating microscope, and the cuts in the skin and testicles are so small that they are almost invisible. Most men are back to work in a day or two. The preliminary results are available immediately, and the full biopsy report is complete in about one week.

If the biopsy shows normal production, meaning there is a blockage, Dr. Goldstein explores where the tubes are blocked using a vasogram, or an X-ray study of the vas deferens. He makes a small incision in the scrotum to expose the vas deferens and then injects contrast dye into the vas or the ejaculatory duct. X-rays of the sperm-carrying tubes can pinpoint where the obstruction lies. He then repairs the blockage with microsurgery at the time of the vasogram.

Not all men with a zero sperm count need a testicle biopsy. If a man has low semen volume and pH, his testicles are normal in size, and his vas deferens can be palpated, then an ultrasound scan can reveal an obstruction in his ejaculatory ducts. This transrectal scan is performed by placing a finger-sized ultrasound probe into the rectum. If a man has normal semen volume and pH, normal testicles, normal vas deferens, and full, firm epididymides, a positive antibody test, and normal FSH, this indicates an obstruction in the epididymis or vas deferens. A biopsy is not necessary, and the next step is microsurgery to correct the blockage and/or aspirate and freeze sperm for future use in IVF with ICSI.

Dr. Goldstein may also use the testicle biopsy to retrieve sperm from the testicles to be used for ICSI, or the biopsied tissue may be frozen and stored for future use in managing infertility.

In the Future

Advanced diagnostic genetic technology will allow us to identify more genes that are associated with infertility. Ultimately, we hope that when a genetic basis is found, gene therapy could offer a cure.

* * * * * * *

A thorough history and physical examination of the male partner is only half of the couple's evaluation. The female partner also needs to be fully evaluated, particularly if the man has antisperm antibodies. A postcoital test to check how well the man's sperm navigates the female partner's cervical mucus is just one of the many tests you can read about in the next chapter.

Take-Home Messages

- The most common cause of male infertility is a varicocele, or enlarged veins in the scrotum.
- The first visit with a fertility specialist should include a detailed medical history, thorough physical examination, semen analysis, and blood tests for hormone levels.
- Know whether your laboratory used standard or stricter (Kruger) criteria to measure sperm morphology, in particular if you need a second opinion or are sharing lab results with another doctor.
- If you have a zero sperm count, you need genetic testing and may require a testicular biopsy.

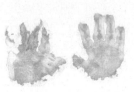

What Tests Should a Woman Have?
A Female Fertility Evaluation

. . . .

"When I first went to see Dr. Rosenwaks, he told me we might have some trouble having a baby because of my age," says Patricia a forty-one-year-old painter. "He asked me, 'How many kids do you want?' I said three. 'Then we have to get to work,' he said."

Dr. Rosenwaks did a full workup on Patricia and did not find any particular fertility issues. Her husband, Jack, a forty-seven-year-old minister, came with her to all of the tests. "I went to as many as I could," says Jack, whose sperm count was on the low side of normal. "When we went in for various tests, including the sonogram to check Patricia's ovaries, we didn't know what to expect. I felt like it would be better if I was there with my wife."

With a diagnosis of unexplained infertility, Jack and Patricia have begun to prepare for their first intrauterine insemination cycle.

. . . .

This chapter describes Dr. Rosenwaks's straightforward approach to the workup of the infertile couple. Briefly, the evaluation endeavors to look at several critical areas involved in human reproduction. These include tests for ovulation; assessment of hormone production, especially the hormones that are critical for supporting embryo implantation and early pregnancy; evaluation of cervical mucus, the uterine cavity, and the fallopian tubes, all necessary for sperm transport, egg and embryo transport, and implantation; sperm function tests, including evaluation of sperm density, movement, and shape; and making sure that the pelvic organs are intact and functioning normally.

As with every other medical assessment, a careful and comprehensive medical history is taken first and is then followed by a complete physical examination. Appropriate tests are scheduled to evaluate the cervix, uterus, and fallopian tubes. Hormonal screening is obtained, including baseline hormone studies for follicle-stimulating hormone (FSH), estrogen, and anti-Müllerian hormone (AMH) in the early follicular phase to assess ovarian reserve, as well as progesterone levels in the second half of the cycle. More specific tests are performed later, depending on the initial findings.

The Female Fertility Evaluation

The first step in the female fertility evaluation is to take a careful history. Certain clues in the history help lead Dr. Rosenwaks to a diagnosis. If a woman has a previous history of sexually transmitted disease, pelvic inflammatory disease (PID), or ruptured appendix or has used an intrauterine device (IUD), her infertility may be due to tubal disease. If she has menstrual irregularities or no periods, milk leaking from her breasts (galactorrhea), or hot flashes, this provides clues to hormonal abnormalities or ovarian dysfunction. A woman with severe pain during menstruation or intercourse may have endometriosis, which is defined as uterine endometrial tissue growing outside the confines of the uterus. When endometriosis is found in the pelvis, it can cause scarring and/or anatomic distortion that may result in infertility.

Initial Consultation

Before seeing a couple, Dr. Rosenwaks asks both partners to complete a background questionnaire that describes their previous fertility history, workup performed, and specifics of previous treatments. When possible, all previous medical records should be sent to him before the initial visit.

The simple questionnaire identifies whether the couple has had any previous in vitro fertilization (IVF) procedure or pelvic surgery. The initial history includes questions about any pregnancies, miscarriages, or ectopic pregnancies. A menstrual history asks about the woman's age of menstrual onset, interval between periods, and length and pattern of her menstrual bleeding. Questions regarding a previous diagnosis of endometriosis, an abnormally shaped uterus, or whether the woman is a "DES daughter" may provide clues to the reason for her infertility. Diethylstilbestrol (DES), a synthetic estrogen, was prescribed during the 1950s and 1960s to prevent miscarriages but was found to cause malformations in the reproductive organs of some women (and men) exposed to it before birth.

A woman's pregnancy history is very important. Dr. Rosenwaks finds out how long the couple has been trying to get pregnant, whether the woman has ever been pregnant, and the results of any pregnancies.

Then he asks about previous procedures to investigate fertility issues. These may include such tests as a hysterosalpingogram, endometrial biopsy, hysteroscopy, or laparoscopy. He notes whether the woman has had any pelvic or abdominal surgery.

A basic history of major medical problems helps identify any conditions that may impair fertility. Major systemic problems can often cause infertility, including uncontrolled or poorly controlled diabetes, thyroid disease, or tuberculosis. Previous cancer therapy may also lead to infertility.

Knowing that infertility often has a male component, Dr. Rosenwaks gathers information about the male partner's reproductive and urologic history. He checks the results of previous semen analyses, asks whether the man has been diagnosed and possibly treated for a varicocele, and discusses any antibiotic treatment for genital tract infections such as chlamydia or mycoplasma. He also investigates the man's history of major medical problems that may affect fertility, such as diabetes, and whether the man is taking medications, including antidepressant drugs such as selective serotonin reuptake inhibitors and other psychotropic medications.

Dr. Rosenwaks discusses the tests both partners may have had during basic fertility workups with other doctors. This includes antisperm antibody tests, which show if the movement of the man's sperm is inhibited by antibodies that are attached to his sperm or found in his or his female partner's blood. Another test that many couples may have is the postcoital test. This is a microscopic examination of a woman's cervical mucus at the fertile time of her cycle to determine the number and motility of her male partner's sperm following intercourse.

Physical Exam

Next, Dr. Rosenwaks conducts a complete physical examination of the female partner. Just as for a man, a woman's body, in particular her hair distribution and breast appearance, may provide hints about fertility issues. If a woman has excessive hair growth, a milky discharge from her breasts, or has not had her period for six months, she is likely to have hormonal problems. Dr. Rosenwaks would then order additional hormone tests as well as imaging studies to pin down the diagnosis.

Female Reproductive Anatomy

(Courtesy Vanessa Dudley)

After the general physical, he does a pelvic exam. This helps him identify any anatomic abnormalities of the uterus, ovaries, and other pelvic organs. He dons surgical gloves and begins the pelvic exam with an examination of the vagina for any discharges. An inflamed vagina or vaginal discharges may indicate an infection. Some simple lab tests can identify whether the inflammation is due to a yeast infection or the parasite trichomonas. These infections can be irritating but generally do not cause infertility.

Genital warts, or condyloma, are caused by an infection with human papilloma virus. Although this virus does not cause PID, it is linked to cervical cancer, and women with genital warts are more likely to have infections with bacteria and other organisms that can lead to infertility.

Then Dr. Rosenwaks undertakes a careful examination of the vagina and cervix for anatomic defects. A vaginal ridge (septum) may suggest that an associated abnormality may be present higher up in the reproductive tract, and a septum in the uterus can be responsible for repeated miscarriages. The presence of uterine abnormalities can be confirmed by X-rays (hysterogram) or a magnetic resonance imaging (MRI) scan.

Adenosis (abnormally placed glandular tissue) in the vagina or cervix may suggest that the patient was exposed to DES before birth. An inflamed cervix that bleeds when touched with a sterile Q-tip may indicate an active infection. Cervical inflammation may lead to scanty or no cervical mucus production and may interfere with the upward migration of sperm into the female reproductive tract.

Dr. Rosenwaks performs an internal exam to evaluate the shape, position, and size of the uterus. If the woman's uterus is fixed (not movable) or tilted backward, and he can feel nodules or thickness in that area, this could indicate that the woman has endometriosis or has had a previous pelvic infection. An enlarged, irregularly shaped uterus could signify that the woman has fibroids.

Normally, the fallopian tubes cannot be felt during a physical exam. Any fullness on either side of the uterus could represent either fluid-filled, obstructed fallopian tubes or enlargement of the ovaries. An ultrasound scan may be useful to confirm the presence of abnormalities of the fallopian tubes or the ovaries. Enlarged ovaries may signify ovarian cysts, endometriosis, or other tumors. Ultrasound examination is critical for confirming the presence of polycystic ovaries, which, when associated with a lack of ovulation and findings of multiple small cysts in the ovaries, confirms the diagnosis of polycystic ovarian syndrome (PCOS).

Finally, he completes the pelvic exam by inserting one finger in the woman's vagina and another into her rectum to feel for thickening of the vaginal septum, which can indicate that she has endometriosis.

Postcoital Test

If the physical exam indicates a potential problem with the woman's cervical mucus, Dr. Rosenwaks performs a postcoital test. A postcoital test is particularly useful for evaluating the interaction between the male partner's sperm and the female partner's cervical mucus. If antisperm antibodies are bound to any region of the sperm, the antibodies will react with the cervical mucus and may prevent the sperm from passing through the cervix. A genital tract infection can cause changes in the cervical mucus that may interfere with sperm penetration or survival.

The timing of the postcoital test is key. The test should be done when the woman's mucus is the most receptive, that is, just before she ovulates. If previous postcoital tests were not timed properly, Dr. Rosenwaks asks the couple to come into his office at the right time to repeat the test. If he sees sperm moving freely in the cervical mucus, that's a good sign that the sperm can make it through the woman's cervical mucus. But if the test reveals only slow-moving or dead sperm, then her cervical mucus may be "hostile" to her male partner's sperm, contributing to poor sperm motility or survival. A postcoital test can be a useful predictor of success of subsequent intrauterine inseminations (IUIs).

If the male partner has a fair-to-good semen analysis, but the postcoital test is poor, then Dr. Rosenwaks may recommend that the couple try IUI. IUI is artificial insemination of sperm, which have been washed free of seminal fluid, directly into the uterus. IUI can overcome cervical mucus problems and decreased sperm counts.

The postcoital test is not used by all fertility experts. Some believe that its usefulness as a diagnostic tool is limited.

Ovulation Assessment

One of the easiest ways to find out when the woman is ovulating is for her to keep a basal body temperature (BBT) chart. Although this method is rarely used today, a rise in temperature in the second half of the cycle is a sign of ovulation. The BBT chart usually shows that a woman's temperature rises by about 0.5°F after ovulation. The rise in BBT is a response to progesterone, which is secreted by the corpus luteum after ovulation.

Home ovulation test kits available in drugstores also allow a woman to detect the surge of luteinizing hormone (LH) that occurs just before she ovulates. Counting the first day of the menstrual period as day one, Dr. Rosenwaks instructs the woman to start testing on day 9 and to keep testing each day until she gets a positive result. Most women with a twenty-eight day cycle ovulate on day 14, but many women have longer or shorter cycles, so you may need to test a few extra days before or after mid-cycle to make sure you note your ovulation day. These home ovulation test kits can also help assure a woman that she is indeed ovulating.

Other signs of ovulation include abundant slippery cervical mucus with the consistency of raw egg whites which disappears with ovulation and a twinge of pain on one side of the lower abdomen. A blood test that shows an elevation in progesterone in the middle of the luteal phase of the menstrual cycle is the best indirect evidence of ovulation.

Ultrasound Scans

An ultrasound scan is an important part of the woman's fertility workup. The ripening follicle produces increasing quantities of estrogen, which cause the endometrium to thicken. The thickness and pattern of the endometrium on the ultrasound scan can give a good idea of how much estrogen a woman is producing. This does not, however, give any indication of the quality of the egg or ovulation.

Ultrasound scans bounce high-frequency sound waves off the pelvic organs. The reflected sound waves are received by the ultrasound probe (transducer), and a computer reconstructs the waves into black-and-white images on a monitor.

The standard ultrasound technique used today is a vaginal ultrasound. Dr. Rosenwaks inserts a long, slender probe into the vagina to image the pelvic organs. This technique is much more comfortable than the older abdominal ultrasound that required you to fill up your bladder to its fullest, and it provides sharper and clearer images because the vaginal probe is much closer to the pelvic structures.

The vaginal ultrasound scan allows Dr. Rosenwaks to determine when one of the woman's follicles has grown and is likely to contain a mature egg. He also can count the number of small follicles within the ovary that may be capable of developing during a stimulation cycle. A woman who has several follicles in each ovary is likely to have a normal ovarian reserve, that is, she has a reasonable number of eggs in her ovary and a good chance of becoming pregnant when she undergoes hormonal stimulation of her ovaries.

The ultrasound scan can also provide clear pictures of the uterus and ovaries. Dr. Rosenwaks can check for small benign tumors embedded in the uterine lining (fibroids, or polyps), and check for ovarian cysts. He can also see whether the fallopian tubes are filled with fluid and can detect an ectopic (tubal) pregnancy. Ultrasound scans can also monitor the early stages of a normal pregnancy.

One of the most common findings on an ultrasound scan is an ovarian cyst. An ovarian cyst is a fluid-filled sac that develops in the ovary. During ovulation, a follicle may grow but fail to rupture and release an egg. Instead of being reabsorbed, the fluid within the follicle forms into a cyst. Or a cyst may develop when the corpus luteum, which develops from the follicle after it has released an egg, fills with blood. These ovarian cysts are not related to disease and usually disappear on their own within sixty days without treatment, although they may delay or reduce the effectiveness of fertility treatments.

Ovarian cysts can occur, however, with some fertility-impairing conditions, such as PCOS, endometriosis (the cysts are called endometriomas), and ovarian tumors. An ultrasound scan can be used to look at these cysts or solid growths within the ovaries. Simple cysts have clear fluid and thin walls. A woman with PCOS has many small, smooth cysts that look like a necklace of pearls. Fluid-filled endometriomas (also called chocolate cysts) look like gray, complex masses. Ultrasound is also used to follow the development of follicles (small egg-containing sacs) during ovulation induction with clomiphene or gonadotropins.

Hormone Screening

Normal ovulation and monthly menstrual cycling require proper functioning of the body's endocrine system. Dr. Rosenwaks routinely conducts blood tests to check a woman's ovarian reserve by measuring day 3 hormone levels of FSH, LH, and estradiol, and when possible, AMH. He makes sure that the thyroid, adrenal, and pituitary hormones are normal.

Thyroid function is evaluated by measuring thyroid stimulating hormone (TSH) and free thyroxine levels in the blood. Women with low thyroid hormone levels may have menstrual disturbances or recurrent miscarriages. Those with high thyroid hormone levels characteristically have a decreased menstrual flow and may not ovulate or menstruate.

Dr. Rosenwaks always measures a fasting prolactin level. If a woman's blood levels of prolactin are high, and she is not taking medication that

Normal Values of Female Hormones

Follicle-stimulating hormone (mIU/ml)		
Early follicular phase		<12
Adult female		3.0–14.4
Postmenopausal female		>40
Luteinizing hormone (mIU/ml)		
Early follicular phase		<10
Mid-cycle surge		>17
Nonovulatory		1.1–11.6
Estradiol (pg/ml)		
Follicular phase		ND–84
Late follicular phase		ND–160
Luteal		27–246
Prolactin (ng/ml)		
Nonpregnant		1.9–25
Progesterone (ng/ml)		
Follicular phase		ND–1.13
Luteal phase		>3.0
17 hydroxyprogesterone (ng/ml)		
Follicular phase		0.10–0.80
Luteal phase		0.27–2.96
Testosterone (ng/ml)		ND–81 ng/dL
Free testosterone		0.9%–3.8%
DHEAS	Adult	80–560 µg/dL
Androstenedione (ng/ml)		1.54–2.34
TSH (mU/L)		0.34–5.60 mIU/ml
		0.4–2.5 (desired range)
Total T4 (µg/dL)		4.5–12.0
Free T4 (ng/dL)		0.6–1.6

< = less than, > = greater than, mIU = milli international units, ml = milliliter,
pg = picograms, ng = nanograms, µIU = micro–international units,
dl = deciliter, mcg = micrograms, ND = nondetectable

Values from the Endocrinology Laboratory at New York Hospital.
Normal values may vary in other laboratories.

increases prolactin, he orders an MRI scan of the pituitary to check for tumors before initiating treatment.

If blood test results show a high LH-to-FSH ratio (more than twice the normal ratio), and the woman has irregular periods, excess hair growth, and a body mass index above 25 (which indicates she's overweight) or her ultrasound scan shows ovarian cysts in the typical "necklace sign," Dr. Rosenwaks suspects she has PCOS. Then he obtains more blood for an androgen panel to measure the male hormones testosterone, free testosterone, androstenedione, and dehydroepiandrosterone sulfate (DHEAS), as well as her 17-hydroxyprogesterone level. According to the results of these tests, he may suspect the woman has a mild version of an inherited disorder that increases production of androgens from the adrenal glands. To diagnose this condition, known as congenital adrenal hyperplasia (or nonclassical adrenal hyperplasia), he orders a stimulation test with an adrenal hormone, adrenocorticotropic hormone.

Levels of FSH, LH, estrogen, and AMH are obtained on the third day of the menstrual cycle to evaluate a woman's ovarian reserve. High FSH levels above 15 to 20 milli–international units per milliliter indicate a profoundly diminished ovarian reserve, especially when a woman's AMH levels are very low. FSH levels above 40 milli–international units per milliliter show that the woman has ovarian failure (or premature menopause).

Most women who have elevated FSH levels and low AMH concentrations on day 3 do not respond well to ovarian stimulating drugs and tend to have a poorer chance of becoming pregnant, particularly if they need assisted reproductive technology treatments. Even a single elevated FSH level in a woman who has fluctuating cycle-to-cycle FSH levels denotes a lower chance for conception with IVF compared to a woman of the same age with normal FSH levels.

Some investigators have used various other tests to evaluate ovarian reserve, especially in women older than age thirty-five. One such test is the clomiphene citrate challenge test (CCCT). This test uses the drug clomiphene citrate (10 mg) from day 3 to day 9. A marked elevation of FSH on day 10 indicates poor ovarian reserve. As this test is not an absolute marker of fertility, the results of this test should not be used to deny treatment. This is also true for all ovarian reserve tests, which provide relative rather than absolute prognostic markers for a woman's fertility potential.

Further Fertility Tests

The results of these initial tests and procedures help guide whether Dr. Rosenwaks needs to perform further tests to find out more about the couple's infertility. These tests involve X-rays, hysteroscopy, laparoscopy, or a biopsy of the uterine lining.

Before performing any of these tests, Dr. Rosenwaks makes sure the woman is free of infections such as chlamydia. If need be, both the woman and her male partner take antibiotic treatments to treat these infections. This will reduce the chance of spreading infection through the woman's reproductive tract during these additional tests.

Hysterosalpingogram

A hysterosalpingogram is an X-ray test that evaluates the shape and contours of the uterus and fallopian tubes. The test can be used to identify abnormalities in the uterus such as adhesions, polyps, or tumors and whether the fallopian tubes are open.

The test is carried out during the first half of the woman's menstrual cycle, after her menstrual flow has stopped but before ovulation. It is important to wait until menstrual bleeding has stopped so that endometrial cells are not pushed through the fallopian tubes into the pelvic cavity, since this could potentially result in endometriosis.

If performed carefully and gently, a hysterosalpingogram causes minimal discomfort. When a woman's cervix is tight, which might cause some discomfort, she can take a mild pain medication such as Advil one hour before the procedure. For the test, an X-ray machine is placed over the woman's abdomen to take pictures of the uterus and fallopian tubes. A small tube is placed through the cervix, and a small amount of radiopaque dye is injected. The dye fills the uterus and moves through the fallopian tubes. If the tubes are open, the dye spills out of the far ends of the tubes. If the tubes are blocked at the far end, they will stretch and balloon out. The dye, which appears white on X-rays, also provides an outline of the uterine cavity.

Sometimes a woman may have stomach cramps for a day or two after the test. She will receive a prescription for a broad-spectrum antibiotic, such as doxycycline, for a few days afterward to prevent any infections.

Just cleaning debris from the fallopian tubes may increase a couple's chances of conceiving, so Dr. Rosenwaks encourages couples to have well-timed intercourse during the cycle when he performs the hysterosalpingogram.

Hysteroscopy

If the hysterosalpingogram suggests that the woman has uterine abnormalities, then a hysteroscopy is performed to confirm the defects. This test helps visualize uterine fibroids, adhesions, a divided or double-shaped uterus, or a T-shaped uterine cavity associated with DES exposure in utero.

The test is usually performed early in the woman's menstrual cycle, before the uterine lining fully develops. This affords a clear view of the uterus. Later in the cycle, the lining thickens and may obscure the view. If he wants to obtain an endometrial biopsy to evaluate the adequacy or level of uterine lining maturation, then Dr. Rosenwaks schedules the hysteroscopy late in the luteal phase of the woman's cycle.

A hysteroscopy can be performed under local anesthesia or with intravenous sedation. A thin fiberoptic device called a hysteroscope is inserted into the uterus through the cervix. Fluid is injected to distend the uterus and reveal the uterine cavity. Abnormalities such as polyps, scars, or tumors (such as fibroids) are documented and, if necessary, surgically removed or corrected with the hysteroscope. This procedure can be used to remove a uterine septum, dissolve intrauterine scars, and remove polyps or submucosal fibroids. The development of safer distension media, better optics, and surgical scissors for the hysteroscope has revolutionized and simplified surgical procedures within the cavity of the uterus.

Laparoscopy

In contrast to hysteroscopy, which is used to visualize the uterine cavity through a tube inserted through the cervix, laparoscopy utilizes a thin, fiber-optic, magnifying instrument to visualize the abdominal and pelvic organs through an incision made near the navel.

At times, laparoscopy is combined with hysteroscopy to ensure that procedures performed on the uterus do not cause perforation or damage. Visualization of the pelvic organs by laparoscopy allows the fertility expert to examine the ovaries, the fallopian tubes, and the surface of the pelvis and of the uterus. This procedure helps the fertility expert to diagnose scarring of the fallopian tubes resulting from PID, endometriosis, pelvic adhesions, ovarian cysts, uterine fibroids, and tubal damage or obstruction.

A laparoscopy is performed under general anesthesia. The laparoscope is a thin fiber-optic instrument with a special camera at one end. After the abdomen is distended with carbon dioxide, a small incision is made at the lower edge of the woman's navel, and the laparoscope is inserted into the abdomen. A second or third instrument may also be inserted into either side of the lower abdomen to move the pelvic organs and to perform any necessary pelvic surgery. The laparoscope is not only used to diagnose pelvic disease; the fertility expert can perform extensive surgery to restore normal anatomy and remove interfering pelvic adhesions.

Nowadays, robotic surgery can be performed through the laparoscope, allowing the fertility expert to accomplish major procedures that previously had to be done through the abdomen with a large incision. An experienced laparoscopic surgeon can perform all repairs and do reconstructive surgery with this minimally invasive approach. This includes removal of endometriosis, repair of fallopian tubes, removal of pelvic adhesions, and ablation (burning) of endometriosis. A laparoscopy not only provides more information about the woman's reproductive anatomy, it provides an opportunity to treat problems immediately.

As with every operation, there is a small risk of bleeding, infection, or damage to vital organs, but laparoscopy is generally safe and effective.

Endometrial Biopsy

In an endometrial biopsy, a small amount of tissue is scraped from the endometrium with a plastic vacuum tube, and this tissue is sent to the pathology laboratory for evaluation. A pathologist checks the tissue and evaluates its development. The endometrial lining undergoes a predictable and orderly development, with typical changes occurring in a clocklike fashion once ovulation occurs and progesterone levels increase. To date the tissue sample properly, the woman must notify Dr. Rosenwaks once her next period starts after the biopsy. A woman's menstrual cycle begins when the endometrium achieves a typical appearance of a day-28 lining. Dr. Rosenwaks can compare the actual date of her cycle with the pathologist's dating of the tissue's development. A biopsy that is three or more days out of phase suggests a luteal phase defect (LPD). The diagnosis can be confirmed by a second biopsy in a subsequent cycle. It should be emphasized that LPD is a rare condition but when present may cause repeated pregnancy loss.

An endometrial biopsy is the gold standard for diagnosing a luteal phase defect; however, multiple progesterone levels can also be good diagnostic substitutes. Progesterone levels obtained on days 5, 7, and 9 after ovulation are used to evaluate progesterone secretion. Generally, if all three levels are lower than 10 nanograms per milliliter, your doctor may need to confirm the diagnosis with an endometrial biopsy.

In the Future

Ultrasound technology has made dramatic advances in recent years and holds promise for assessing whether fallopian tubes are open, visualizing blood flow through the pelvis, and identifying uterine abnormalities.

Advances in Ultrasound

Ultrasound tests now allow doctors to assess whether fallopian tubes are open without having to use X-rays. This test, called sonosalpingography, can show whether the fallopian tubes are normal. The test involves passing a fluid into the woman's tubes through the uterus to see the passage of bubbles into the tubes and out into the abdomen. However, the gold standard for testing the fallopian tubes is still a hysterosalpingogram and laparoscopy, because the doctor can visualize them directly and more accurately.

New ultrasound machines may have attachments that allow the doctor to watch the flow of blood. A color Doppler ultrasound scan allows the doctor to visualize the blood in color as it flows through the pelvic blood vessels. This is still being evaluated for its clinical usefulness.

Three-dimensional (3-D) ultrasound machines use sophisticated microprocessors that reconstruct an image of the internal organs and provide a 3-D view. This is useful to help a doctor, for example, differentiate between a divided uterus (septate) and a heart-shaped one. The pictures allow visualization of internal organs in 3-D, but the true value of 3-D ultrasound technology for infertility needs to be further validated.

. . . .

After Drs. Rosenwaks and Goldstein have completed their evaluations of both partners, they devise a treatment plan for the couple. The next two chapters describe the standard treatments for both male and female infertility.

Take-Home Messages

- A background questionnaire provides the fertility specialist with information about your previous fertility history, any workups you may have had, and specific information about previous treatments.
- A complete and careful physical examination can provide clues about your possible fertility problems.
- A postcoital test should be performed when your mucus is at the most fertile stage—just before you ovulate.
- Home ovulation test kits can help show when you are ovulating.
- Day 3 levels of FSH, LH, estrogen, and AMH help determine your ovarian reserve.
- A hysterosalpingogram can evaluate the shape and contours of your uterus and fallopian tubes, as well as whether the tubes are open.
- A hysteroscopy can confirm and treat defects in your uterus.
- A laparoscopy can diagnose abdominal and pelvic problems and also remove or burn away endometriosis, repair fallopian tubes, and remove pelvic adhesions.
- An endometrial biopsy is the gold standard for diagnosing a luteal phase defect, which is a rare condition.

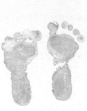

Eight

Taking Action for Men
Male Infertility Causes and Treatments

*H*istorically, infertility has been considered a woman's disease. It's only within the last fifty years that the importance of the male contribution to infertility has been recognized. In fact, in at least half of all infertility cases, a male factor is either the main or a significant contributing cause. The mistaken notion that infertility is associated with impotence or decreased masculinity may have contributed to men's reluctance to be tested.

The good news is that the rapid research advances in the area of male reproduction have brought about dramatic changes in the ability both to diagnose and to treat male infertility. The majority of couples in which the man suffers from male infertility can now be helped to conceive a child on their own.

Varicocele Repair

. . . .

After years of trying to start a family, Steve and Rachel's fears began to give way to hopelessness. "Nothing was happening, so we decided to check things out, to see if everything was okay with me and with him," recalls Rachel, who was then a thirty-three-year-old homemaker. Her husband, Steve, who was then a thirty-three-year old computer expert, went to see a urologist, and the results were not good. "My sperm count and testosterone levels were low," recalls Steve. "We were devastated. We didn't think we would be able to have children."

Steve's urologist recommended that he see Dr. Goldstein. He found that Steve had large varicoceles that surrounded both of his testicles, which heated them up and caused his poor sperm count and low testosterone levels. Dr. Goldstein performed microsurgery with minimal anesthesia in an outpatient procedure to tie off and eliminate these varicose veins. Steve's sperm function and testosterone levels improved, and this allowed Rachel to conceive.

. . . .

As discussed above, the most common identifiable cause of infertility in men is a varicocele. Just over one third of infertile men who have never fathered a child have a varicocele, and 80 percent of men who were once fertile but are now infertile also have a varicocele. Varicoceles are abnormally enlarged veins draining the testicles. They cause pooling of blood in the scrotum and a rise in testicular temperature. Even a one-degree rise in temperature in the scrotum can have an adverse effect on sperm production and testosterone function.

The good news is that varicoceles are treatable. Dozens of reports have been published demonstrating the benefit of varicocele surgery to improve sperm counts. Yet varicocele repair remains controversial, particularly for small varicoceles that can't be seen or felt on a physical exam. Studies have shown greater improvements in semen quality for repair of large varicoceles compared with smaller ones.

Microscopes were not used in older surgical procedures to repair varicoceles, which made it extremely difficult to locate the tiny artery that provides the major source of nourishment for the testicles. This artery was often tied off, which interfered with testicular function. Tiny lymph ducts were also inadvertently tied off, often causing a condition called hydrocele, which is a bag of fluid that develops around the testicle.

These results led Dr. Goldstein to develop a microsurgical technique of varicocele repair using an operating microscope. This enabled him to identify and preserve the main artery and the lymph ducts, eliminating the potential for damage to the testicle as well as virtually eliminating the complication of hydrocele. With the use of this technique in several thousand patients, the average healthy sperm count after repair of large varicoceles has been shown to increase 128 percent. Dr. Goldstein can help couples achieve a 43 percent pregnancy rate one year after surgery and a 69 percent pregnancy rate after two years with microscopic varicocele surgery. This compares to only a 17 percent pregnancy rate after one year in couples if the man declined surgery.

Microsurgical varicocele repair takes about one hour for each testicle. The procedure is performed with the man asleep under light general anesthesia or awake with a regional anesthetic (spinal or epidural) that makes him completely numb from the waist down. The total time in the operating room is about three hours if both sides are done. This includes time for skin shaving, anesthesia before the operation, bandaging, and awakening from anesthesia after the surgery.

Most men feel some discomfort for the first two to three weeks after the surgery. Dr. Goldstein provides a prescription for pain medication. Swelling and bruising of the penis and scrotum are normal and take about three weeks to completely resolve. He also suggests the man apply ice to the incision for forty-eight hours postoperatively to help decrease pain and swelling.

There are no stitches to remove. The stitching is beneath the skin and dissolves by itself. All the man has to do is remove tiny strips of tape, called Steri-Strips, ten days after the operation. He can resume sex in one week and all normal activities after three weeks.

One month after the surgery, Dr. Goldstein sees the man to check on his recovery. At three months, the man has a semen analysis or postcoital test, and another semen analysis or postcoital test at six months, and again every six months until his female partner becomes pregnant.

Microsurgical repair of varicoceles improves semen quality and quantity and testosterone levels with less postoperative pain compared to a nonmicrosurgical technique. Yet most urologists who perform varicocele repairs do not use a microscope. Varicoceles can also be repaired with conventional surgery without a microscope, with surgery through a laparoscope, or with balloon occlusion that uses small silicone spheres to block off the enlarged veins.

Varicocele repair has another important function. The testicles have two purposes: one is the production of the sperm, and the other is to produce testosterone. Dr. Goldstein's research shows the presence of varicoceles causes significantly lower testosterone levels, and following varicocele repair, testosterone levels are greatly improved in more than two thirds of men

Unblocking Ducts

The second major cause of infertility in men is blockages or obstructions along the male reproductive tract. This is particularly true for men with zero sperm count, a condition called azoospermia. Men with zero sperm counts can be divided into two broad groups: men who have an obstruction or blockage, meaning they are making sperm, but the sperm can't get out; and men who have a sperm production problem, meaning they are not making sperm, a condition called nonobstructive azoospermia (NOA). Dr. Goldstein can usually determine which group an infertile male falls into by examining him and doing blood tests for follicle stimulating hormone (FSH), testosterone, and genetic tests. If a man has smaller-than-normal testicles, an elevated FSH, or an abnormal genetic test, Dr. Goldstein knows it is NOA. If a man has normal testicles, swollen ducts, and a positive anti-sperm antibody test, he knows it is a blockage. If these tests are inconclusive, then he performs a testicular biopsy to evaluate whether the testicles are producing sperm; he uses a microscope, which minimizes discomfort and complications.

Typically, blockages are caused by a urinary tract infection or by the sexually transmitted diseases chlamydia and gonorrhea. Bacteria can infect the epididymis, which is essentially a swimming school for sperm before they are able to fertilize an egg. Infection of the epididymis can cause scarring and blockage, inhibiting the sperm from leaving this tiny duct.

With the use of microscopes, Dr. Goldstein can repair epididymal blockages successfully up to 90 percent of the time. Sperm reappear in the ejaculate in 90 percent of men, and 40 percent will father a child. Also during surgery, if he finds sperm in the fluid of the epididymis, he aspirates (suctions out) the sperm and freezes them. All it takes is a few good sperm for a possible future intracytoplasmic sperm injection (ICSI) procedure, which injects a single sperm directly into an egg.

Another potential cause of blocked ducts is hernia repair. Up to 17 percent of men who have surgery to repair a hernia end up with a blocked vas deferens. Usually only one testicle is damaged, but if both testicles have had hernia repairs or the one functioning testicle is damaged, the man could end up infertile. Dr. Goldstein can microsurgically repair the blocked ducts and help more than half of these men impregnate their female partners.

Vasectomy Reversal

. . . .

"I was married previously and I had had a vasectomy," says Gary, a forty-eight-year-old businessman. "When Betty and I married, we wanted the option to have children. I had a vasectomy reversal, but it didn't work." So Gary and his wife Betty, age forty-two, a schoolteacher, did some research. "We heard Dr. Goldstein's name several times from people in the field," says Gary.

They met with Dr. Goldstein, who explained how he would use microsurgery to reconnect Gary's tiny sperm-carrying tubes that had previously been cut. "I was surprised at how quickly I recovered from the surgery and how little pain I felt," says Gary.

"We were thrilled when the procedure worked," adds Betty. Now the couple has a four-and-a-half-year-old daughter.

. . . .

One of the most common causes of blockage is a vasectomy. Approximately half a million to one million men undergo vasectomy each year in the United States for permanent birth control. With an increase in divorce rates coast-to-coast, the demand for vasectomy reversal is also growing. Men typically seek to reverse a vasectomy for one of three reasons: they have remarried, they have lost a child, or they have had a change of heart.

Using a precise microsurgical technique he developed, Dr. Goldstein achieves return of sperm in more than 99 percent of men undergoing vasectomy reversal if he finds sperm in at least one of their vas ducts. Within one year, 70 percent of the female partners of these men become pregnant.

Much as an architect prepares blueprints before the builder constructs the house, Dr. Goldstein meticulously plans the placement of sutures during a vasectomy reversal. This painstaking planning allows him to focus on one task at the time of suture placement—hitting the bull's-eye. Using a microtip tissue-marking pen, he maps out the points where his tiny needle will enter and exit. He then reattaches the vas deferens by lining up the dots with six sutures for each of the inner, middle, and outer layers of the vas to secure a leak-proof reconnection.

The outpatient procedure takes three to five hours. The postoperative care and recovery are similar to that for a varicocele repair, although Dr. Goldstein recommends a wait of four weeks before ejaculation in order to avoid disturbing the delicate reconnection of the vas. At the time of the three-month-postoperative semen analysis, he also obtains blood to look for antisperm antibodies that often develop after a vasectomy. In general, it takes from three to twelve months for sperm counts to return to normal, although it can take up to two years.

For men who had a vasectomy less than fifteen years ago, a vasectomy reversal will result in a much higher pregnancy rate than sperm aspiration and an ICSI procedure. Even at intervals greater than fifteen years, reversal outcomes will equal or exceed those of ICSI. A man who waits more than fifteen years since his vasectomy may need a more extensive reversal operation that connects the vas deferens to the epididymis to restore his fertility. The success rate for return of sperm drops to 80 percent if both sides need to be reconnected in this more extensive procedure. Dr. Goldstein routinely aspirates and freezes sperm at the time of surgery for a future ICSI procedure in the event the tubes cannot be reconnected successfully.

In addition, vasectomy reversal may be a more cost-effective option than ICSI, especially for couples seeking more than one child. ICSI typically costs more than a vasectomy reversal, which is more likely to be covered by health insurance than is ICSI.

Approximately 1 percent of all infertile men are born with congenital absence of the vas deferens, the equivalent of a vasectomy. Unfortunately, there are no artificial tubes strong enough to replace the vas deferens. However, we are now able to help almost all such men conceive using an operating microscope to retrieve sperm from the tiny ducts of the epididymis, freeze them, and use them later in an ICSI procedure.

Treating Zero Sperm Count

The most exciting new development in the field of male infertility is the ability to treat men with NOA. Even though these men may have no sperm in their semen, we can now find sperm between the cells of the testicles in about half of the men using a technique called microdissection testicular sperm extraction (TESE). Working together, the Weill Cornell team has been able to achieve a 43 percent pregnancy rate in the partners of these men if sperm is found within their testicles.

Genetic testing has revealed that 10 percent to 15 percent of men with NOA are missing a tiny piece of their Y chromosome. This condition is called micro Y deletion. Most human beings have forty-six chromosomes; males have one X chromosome and one Y chromosome, and females have two X chromosomes. The Y chromosome carries the genes that are responsible for producing sperm. Men who have a zero or very low sperm count might be missing a small piece of that Y chromosome. We can help men with micro Y deletion have children through ICSI, but their male children will have the same infertility problem as they do. However, their children will be healthy in every other way. About 5 percent of men with NOA have an extra X chromosome, called Klinefelter syndrome. Using microdissection TESE, sperm can be found in 60 percent of these men. When using sperm found in Klinefelter men, an additional procedure called preimplantation genetic diagnosis (PGD) can be performed on the embryos so that only normal embryos with forty-six chromosomes are transferred into the female partner.

Hormone Therapy

Correcting imbalances of hormones with drug therapy is one of the mainstays in inducing a woman to ovulate, but there is a paucity of medical therapy available for men to improve sperm production or quality. Some drugs may be helpful in carefully selected instances.

Both clomiphene citrate (Clomid) and tamoxifen (Nolvadex) block estrogen receptors and therefore prevent the important negative feedback of estrogens to the hypothalamus and pituitary. These drugs can stimulate gonadotropin-releasing hormone (GnRH) and the release of luteinizing hormone (LH) and follicle-stimulating hormone (FSH). Since FSH is important for sperm production, it is possible that increased FSH in the blood may enhance sperm production.

Clomiphene can increase testosterone levels and sperm density, but there is no evidence that clomiphene treatments help men impregnate their partners. Dr. Goldstein always makes sure his patients are aware of these minimal benefits and the possible, although minimal, risks prior to treatment. Common side effects of clomiphene include visual disturbances, weight gain or loss, changes in libido, gastrointestinal or neurological disturbances, and skin changes.

Tamoxifen can increase sperm density and sperm motility in men with low sperm counts who have normal hormone levels, but the drug seems to have no effect on men with high FSH and LH levels. Combining testosterone with tamoxifen can slightly enhance the drug's effects on sperm; however, testosterone alone suppresses sperm formation and is never used as a solo therapy.

Aromatase inhibitors, such as anastrozole (Arimidex) or testolactone (Teslac), block the conversion of testosterone to estrogen. Treatment with an aromatase inhibitor decreases estrogen levels, which leads to increased LH and FSH release from the pituitary and a subsequent stimulation of the testicles to increase testosterone production. Aromatase inhibitors may play a role in men with high estrogen levels to increase testosterone and lower estrogen production and to improve their sperm counts and sperm motility. Research has shown that men with Klinefelter syndrome may also benefit from treatment with testolactone.

High prolactin levels inhibit production of LH and FSH, which in turn leads to lowered sperm counts, low testosterone levels, and low sex drive. Men with high prolactin levels, commonly due to pituitary tumors or hypothalamus disorders, can take bromocriptine (Parlodel) or cabergoline (Dostinex) to reduce prolactin levels to normal. Bromocriptine appears to increase FSH levels, and this often restores testosterone production and fertility. These drugs can also shrink pituitary tumors.

Other causes of increased prolactin, such as hypothyroidism or drug-induced high prolactin levels, should be treated specifically. A man with low thyroid hormone levels as well as low levels of LH, FSH, and testosterone and low sperm counts and poor sperm motility can be treated with thyroid replacement therapy. This is often the only treatment he needs to restore his fertility.

Hypogonadotropic Hypogonadism

One condition that certainly benefits from hormone treatments is hypogonadotropic hypogonadism. This condition is due to the lack of GnRH production, and if the man has little or no sense of smell, that indicates Kallmann syndrome. If a man has very low or undetectable blood levels of LH,

FSH, and testosterone and has a lack of secondary sexual characteristics, Dr. Goldstein makes the diagnosis of hypogonadotropic hypogonadism.

The most often used treatment for the development of secondary sexual characteristics and maintenance of libido is Depo-Testosterone injections. But to induce sperm formation, the man must stop taking testosterone. Instead, he takes human chorionic gonadotropin (hCG) injections three times a week for three to six months until his blood levels of testosterone become normal, and then human menopausal gonadotropin (hMG) or recombinant FSH (Follistin or Gonal-F) is added to the injection three times a week. Sperm usually begin to appear in his ejaculate from six to 18 months after initiation of therapy. Testicle size and sperm counts remain lower than normal, but pregnancies occur regularly with sperm densities in a range of 2 to 6 million per milliliters. Men who don't respond to gonadotropin replacement may respond to pulses of GnRH administered via a pump.

Specific Medical Treatments

Certain problems can be treated with specific therapies that are as simple as antibiotics for genital tract infections, corticosteroids for antisperm antibodies, or adrenaline-like drugs such as Sudafed (used for common colds) for retrograde ejaculation. Other men who cannot ejaculate due to nerve damage need a specialized medical procedure called electroejaculation to obtain sperm.

Infection

Men who have more than 1 million white blood cells in their sperm may have a genital tract infection, commonly chlamydia or gonorrhea. If a man demonstrates symptoms of a genital tract infection or if his sperm clump together, then Dr. Goldstein obtains semen cultures. Before the cultures, the man cleans his penis, scrotum, and the area just under the scrotum with an antibacterial scrub to avoid contamination with other bacteria.

If the cultures are positive, then Dr. Goldstein prescribes treatment with an antibiotic appropriate for the cultured organism, such as fluoroquinolone or tetracycline, for both partners. If the culture is negative, but Dr. Goldstein has a high clinical suspicion of an infection, he prescribes fluoroquinolone or tetracycline therapy for three to six weeks, treating both partners.

If medical therapy fails, then the man's sperm can be washed, separated from the seminal fluid, and then used for artificial insemination.

Antisperm Antibodies

Dr. Goldstein's approach to the management of patients with antisperm antibodies is to identify and treat the underlying problem, that is, to use microsurgery to correct any obstructions in ducts or any varicoceles to prevent further production of antisperm antibodies. If the female partner has sperm antibodies, she needs to be treated as well. Intrauterine insemination (IUI) is often effective in cases of antibodies in the woman.

If the production of antisperm antibodies cannot be treated with microsurgery, Dr. Goldstein prescribes 20 milligrams of the steroid prednisone for the man and also twice daily for the first ten days of his partner's cycle and 5 milligrams on days 11 through the end of her cycle for three months. Then he reevaluates for the presence of antisperm antibodies. Steroids can produce significant side effects, including ulcers, mood changes, altered glucose metabolism, impaired testicular function, and, very rarely, damage to the bones of the hip, so he follows the couple closely.

If the problem persists, Dr. Goldstein recommends an ICSI procedure, which is highly effective in cases of severe antisperm antibodies on sperm.

Retrograde Ejaculation

A very small number of men with very low or no semen volume ejaculate backward toward the bladder. This retrograde ejaculation, which is often the first symptom of diabetes, is due to nerve damage in the bladder neck. Dr. Goldstein confirms the diagnosis by examining a urine specimen for sperm immediately after the man has ejaculated.

Treatment consists of medications to facilitate closing of the bladder neck during ejaculation. About 25 percent of men will start to ejaculate normally after taking 120 milligrams of pseudoephedrine (Sudafed) three times daily. Dr. Goldstein also recommends that these men try to ejaculate with a full bladder, which may also stimulate the bladder neck to close.

If these measures fail, then he collects sperm from the bladder after ejaculation to be used in IUI or with ICSI.

Electroejaculation

Men with neurologic impairments who cannot ejaculate are candidates for electroejaculation. This would include men with traumatic spinal cord injury (SCI), multiple sclerosis, or diabetes or those who have had surgery to remove abdominal lymph nodes (often to treat testicular cancer). The electroejaculation procedure has been proven to be a safe, effective means to obtain sperm suitable for IUI or in vitro fertilization (IVF).

Electroejaculation is normally performed under general anesthesia, though a man with a complete SCI may not need anesthesia. The procedure begins by first catheterizing the man and emptying his bladder completely. After the urine is drained out, Dr. Goldstein instills a sperm-nourishing medium into the bladder to protect any sperm that may be ejaculated back into the bladder, which frequently occurs.

The patient is placed on his side, and Dr. Goldstein gently inserts into his rectum a well-lubricated probe that has electrodes attached. He then delivers waves of electricity through the probe, increasing the voltage progressively, until the man ejaculates into a cup. Dr. Goldstein catheterizes the man's bladder again to extract any sperm from retrograde ejaculation, which is sent along with the ejaculate to the IVF laboratory for processing. Using this technique, Dr. Goldstein can obtain semen in more than 90 percent of neurologically impaired men, and more than 40 percent of couples subsequently achieve pregnancy with IUI or IVF/ICSI.

A handheld penile vibrator may also allow some couples to obtain sperm with vibratory stimulation in the comfort of their own homes, especially in men with high spinal cord injuries. The man uses the device to stimulate the underside of his penis for a few minutes until he ejaculates. Then he brings the collected semen sample to the Weill Cornell laboratory for processing and insemination into his female partner or for use with IVF. There's a risk of inducing high blood pressure with electroejaculation or the penile vibrator, so the man must practice this technique in Dr. Goldstein's office before he tries it at home. Men who undergo electroejaculation or vibratory stimulation may develop high blood pressure because of a condition called autonomic hyperreflexia. Taking nifedipine beforehand can prevent this complication.

Impotence

Impotence, or erectile dysfunction, affects an estimated 15 to 20 million men in their lifetimes. About 10 percent of men who are unable to achieve or maintain an erection have psychological issues, such as depression, stress, or anxiety. In about 90 percent of men, the cause is disease, such as diabetes, kidney disease, or alcoholism, which can impair blood flow to the penis. In fact, most impotence is due to vascular disease. In addition, prescription drugs, such as antidepressants, high-blood-pressure medication, tranquilizers, and narcotics, can also lead to impotence. Men who have had radiation therapy, a pelvic injury, or pelvic surgery may also find themselves dealing with chronic erectile dysfunction. And a man's lifestyle may also predispose him toward impotence if he uses cocaine or marijuana, smokes cigarettes, or drinks a lot of coffee or alcohol.

Medical Therapy

Psychological counseling or sex therapy is the recommended treatment for men with psychological impotence. One out of four infertile men perceive themselves as "less of a man," and men suffering impotence are often unwilling to discuss their problem. Sex therapy can help men deal with their impotence and ease communications about sexual dysfunction with their partners.

Drug therapy with sildenafil (Viagra), vardenafil (Levitra), or tadalafil (Cialis) has become the initial medical treatment for impotence. These pills block certain enzymes and allow the proper blood flow necessary for an erection. If one pill doesn't work, try a different one to find the best one for you.

These drugs do have side effects, including headache, diarrhea, blurred vision, "blue" vision, and increased light sensitivity. And men who take heart drugs containing nitrate, such as nitroglycerin for chest pains, should avoid taking these drugs, since the combination may cause dangerous drops in blood pressure. Originally there were concerns that these drugs caused an increased risk of heart attack or death due to cardiovascular disease, but the American College of Cardiology and the American Heart Association now both agree that these drugs are safe for men who are not taking nitrate-containing medications.

Two methods can deliver drugs to dilate blood vessels and increase blood flow through the penis. A man can place small suppositories containing prostaglandin E1, a chemical found throughout the body, into his urethra. Or he can inject prostaglandin E1, papaverine, a chemical derived from papaya, or a combination of medications called Trimix into his penis. In rare instances these repeat injections produce scarring inside the penis, leaving a penile implant as the man's only option.

Penile Implants

Penile implants, or prosthetic devices for the penis, are the most common type of surgical procedure for impotence. A penile implant is a particularly good option for those men for whom medical therapy has failed or who have a severe blood-vessel problem that causes their impotence.

The simplest implants consist of malleable semirigid or rigid silicone rods. Inflatable implants consist of hollow tubes implanted into the penis and a pump located in the scrotum. A reservoir of liquid is placed behind the bladder. A squeeze of the reservoir leads to an erection, and a squeeze of a release valve deflates the device. These more sophisticated prostheses require general anesthesia, a hospital stay, and more extensive surgery than a malleable device. Inflatable devices last about fifteen years before needing replacement.

A Nonmedical Option

A noninvasive way of achieving an erection is to use a penile vacuum pump along with a constriction ring. The man places his penis inside a vacuum tube and pumps the air out. The tube sits right up against the base of his penis in order to create a seal and allows blood to flow into his penis. Once the penis becomes erect, he places a rubber ring around the base of the penis to prevent the blood from leaving, then removes the vacuum tube. This therapy can treat many erectile problems, but the device can be quite cumbersome to use.

Vascular Surgery

Vascular reconstructive surgery can also improve the flow of blood within the penis to help a man achieve an erection. If ultrasound tests reveal that a man's penile arteries are blocked or damaged, he may be a candidate for a penile microsurgical revascularization procedure. The best candidates for this procedure are young, otherwise healthy men who have had trauma that damaged their penile arteries. Up to 50 percent of these carefully selected men have their potency restored after surgery.

Some men have good blood flow into the penis, but a leaky vein inside the penis causes them to lose an erection quickly. Dye is injected into the penis to check where the leak is, and the leaky vein is tied off. After surgery, up to 70 percent of men with this problem become potent again.

The potential long-term side effects of both of these surgical procedures are damage to nerves and scar tissue, which can itself cause impotence.

Premature Ejaculation

Another common sexual dysfunction found among men with infertility is premature ejaculation. Between 50 percent and 75 percent of men with infertility report having problems maintaining an erection long enough to ejaculate. Sex therapy and medical therapy may solve this problem.

Sex therapy can help couples with emotional issues about sex and also teach "stop-start" techniques that help men learn to control ejaculation.

Selective serotonin reuptake inhibitors (SSRIs), such as sertraline (Zoloft), paroxetine (Paxil), or fluoxetine (Prozac), can be effective in treating premature ejaculation because one of the side effects of these drugs is to delay ejaculation. A low dose of an SSRI several hours before sexual intercourse may be enough to improve a man's symptoms. Some of the other side effects of these antidepressants are nausea, dry mouth, drowsiness, and decreased libido.

However, SSRIs may have a negative impact on semen quality. Studies at Weill Cornell have shown that SSRIs can reduce semen volume and increase sperm DNA fragmentation (small breaks in the sperm chromosomes). They should be used cautiously in men trying to impregnate their partners.

The man can use a topical anesthetic cream applied to his penis to delay ejaculation. These creams contain lidocaine or prilocaine and can dull sensations on the penis. The man applies the cream just before intercourse and wipes it off when his penis has lost enough sensation to delay ejaculation, which can take up to forty-five minutes, and puts on a condom to protect his partner from genital numbness. However, some men and women say that using these creams reduces their genital sensitivity and their sexual pleasure.

As long as the man is capable of ejaculating, the couple may also use artificial insemination to achieve a pregnancy.

In the Future

Scanning the testicles with powerful Doppler ultrasound may help locate viable sperm. A new topical spray may be able to treat premature ejaculation. And stem cells derived from a man's own testicles, skin, or bone marrow may one day be able to be used to create new sperm.

Doppler Ultrasound

Steady advances in molecular biological techniques have identified more and more genetic defects associated with infertility, especially NOA. These studies have already yielded useful information to predict which men are likely to have sperm found in their testicles.

Powerful micro-Doppler ultrasound shows promise for identifying where to look for sperm in the testicles of men with NOA. Color Doppler ultrasound is proving somewhat predictive of which men may respond best to microsurgical varicocele repair. Dr. Goldstein obtains a color Doppler ultrasound for men with an easily palpable left-side varicocele when he is uncertain whether they have a varicocele on the right side. After a physical exam, he might suspect a second varicocele, but due to a tight scrotum or obesity, he can't quite tell. He recommends varicocele repair for easily palpable varicoceles or in men with tight scrotums who have large varicoceles found by ultrasound.

Aerosol Spray for Premature Ejaculation

An experimental spray-on anesthetic may be a convenient way to prevent premature ejaculation. The aerosol spray contains the same two drugs, lidocaine and prilocaine, found in the cream used by some couples to delay ejaculation. In a study of three hundred men with a history of premature ejaculation, most of them in their thirties, European researchers found that a spray containing the two drugs extended the time to orgasm by more than six times compared to a placebo spray.

The spray is absorbed only by the glans penis, the most sensitive part of the organ, and not by the shaft. It is quickly absorbed, so there is no danger of it rubbing off on the woman, and it acts in five minutes. That gives it a distinct advantage over the anesthetic cream, which needs to be washed off before intercourse and used with a condom, making this technique not useful for couples trying to get pregnant.

The drug spray has been submitted for approval by the Food and Drug Administration and should be available soon.

Stem Cells

Recent research in animals and humans indicates that human stem cells can be harvested from a man's testicles, skin, or bone marrow. Sperm derived from these stem cells can then be injected into his partner's eggs using IVF with ICSI.

Investigators at Weill Cornell have been able to clone sperm in mice. Pups have been successfully conceived and born using this technique in mice. In humans, rare spermlike cells have been created but not yet used to fertilize human eggs. It is likely that this will be successfully done within the next five to ten years. This would offer hope to men who produce no sperm or have lost their testicles to cancer or trauma.

Take-Home Messages

- Varicocele repair can improve your sperm count and greatly improve your testosterone level.
- Microsurgery to reverse a vasectomy leads to a return of sperm in virtually all cases.
- Even if you have a zero sperm count, you may have sperm in the tubules of your testicles that can be retrieved and used in IVF with ICSI.
- Hormone treatments for men are effective in only select instances.
- Sometimes the best therapy is a simple one, for example, antibiotics for genital-tract infections or a common cold remedy for retrograde ejaculation.
- Most men can be successfully treated for impotence with oral medications, penile injections, or penile implants.
- Sex therapy or medical therapy can usually solve the problem of premature ejaculation.

Nine

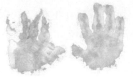

Taking Action for Women

Female Infertility Causes and Treatments

· · · · · · · · · ·

Mary, a thirty-five-year-old clothing saleswoman, and her husband, Ron, a forty-year-old real estate agent, were trying unsuccessfully to get pregnant. Dr. Rosenwaks found some fibroids on Mary's uterus, which he removed surgically through a laparoscope. Ron's sperm count was low due to a varicocele, which Dr. Goldstein repaired. Six months later, Ron's sperm count was still low, and he had antisperm antibodies on his sperm, so Dr. Rosenwaks suggested they try intrauterine insemination (IUI).

Mary took clomiphene to stimulate her ovaries to produce more eggs, but she didn't seem to respond to the drug, so Dr. Rosenwaks switched her to gonadotropin injections. "I mixed the medicine for all of the shots; she gave herself the shots," says Ron. "For the progesterone shots I did both." Mary's ovaries responded, but she did not get pregnant in three tries.

"When you have to come back month after month, you start to get discouraged," Mary says. Ron agrees: "You have to keep giving more sperm samples, and it just wears you out. Dr. Rosenwaks told us to hang in there, that it would work, and to try not to let the disappointments get to us." With their fourth IUI attempt, Mary became pregnant, and their son James is now fifteen months old.

· · · · · · · · · ·

One of the distinct advantages of being evaluated at Weill Cornell is the availability of world-class expertise in both male and female infertility. Couples with infertility often have more than one issue that contributes to their fertility problem, and we specialize in treating couples who have both female- and male-factor problems. Once a couple has gone through fertility evaluations, changed their lifestyles, and attempted basic treatments, all to no avail, there is still hope for them; aggressive medical and surgical approaches enable more than four out of five infertile couples to fulfill their dreams of having a baby—provided that they are willing to undergo all available treatment avenues.

After the reasons for a woman's infertility are identified, Weill Cornell doctors set out to correct the specific cause. This includes hormonal treatments to induce ovulation and medical or surgical treatments to correct endometriosis or anatomical defects. Surgical procedures to correct problems of the fallopian tubes or uterus can be performed as outpatient procedures. When a borderline male factor exists, washing sperm, increasing the fraction of swimming sperm, and placing the sperm directly into the woman's uterus can increase the odds of conception for some couples. Treatment of repeated miscarriages requires identification of the cause and treatment with either medical or surgical therapy. It is especially important to point out that the inability to conceive or maintain a pregnancy is a medical condition that requires careful evaluation and specific treatments aimed at correcting the underlying cause.

Hormone Therapy

An imbalance in reproductive hormones is a frequent cause of infertility. Dr. Rosenwaks utilizes various hormone treatments to correct the hormone flow or to time exactly when to release an egg to optimize fertilization. Once the woman becomes pregnant, hormones can help support the pregnancy. In addition, medication can be used as adjuncts to treat endometriosis, uterine fibroids, and pituitary tumors.

Ovulation Induction

The development of follicles and release of an egg involves a complex interaction between pituitary hormones—follicle-stimulating hormone (FSH) and luteinizing hormone (LH)—and feedback from the ovaries. Normally, a single, mature follicle develops and releases an egg in each menstrual cycle as smaller follicles wither and disappear.

However, this natural flow of hormones can become altered and may prevent a woman from ovulating. FSH and LH secretion may be too low, LH levels may be too high, or the ovaries may function poorly.

Fertility experts now have several hormone medications available to help induce ovulation. Dr. Rosenwaks often uses clomiphene (Clomid), human menopausal gonadotropins (hMG), purified urinary or recombinant FSH, and, rarely, a version of gonadotropin-releasing hormone (GnRH) that can be administered via a pump in a pulsing manner. Agents that may be added to these therapies include dexamethasone and metformin (Glucophage).

Clomiphene

If a woman has not been able to get pregnant because of ovulation problems, clomiphene can increase her chances of conceiving naturally. Clomiphene is a weak estrogen-like drug that binds to estrogen receptors. This fools the brain into thinking that estrogen levels in the blood are too low. The brain tells the hypothalamus to increase pulses of GnRH, which in turn releases more FSH and LH from the pituitary. This stimulates the ovaries to develop more follicles. Typically, clomiphene treatment produces one or two mature follicles each cycle.

Dr. Rosenwaks prescribes clomiphene for five days in a starting dose of 50 milligrams per day, beginning on day 5 of a natural or induced menstrual cycle. In a woman who does not ovulate, it is often advantageous to shed the endometrial lining with a progesterone withdrawal bleed before starting clomiphene. Progesterone is administered for seven to ten days to allow for proper endometrial shedding.

A woman usually ovulates five to ten days after taking the last dose of clomiphene. If she doesn't ovulate, the dose may be adjusted in the next cycle by increasing either the clomiphene dose or the duration of clomiphene treatment. Dr. Rosenwaks prefers to increase the duration of clomiphene to seven days in the first adjusted cycle. If the woman does not ovulate in one more attempt, then he prescribes a 100-milligram dose of clomiphene. Because low-dose injectable gonadotropin (in the form of FSH) regimens work so well in these women, we no longer continue clomiphene treatment for many months. This low-dose gonadotropin regimen will be described later in this chapter.

Half of the women treated with clomiphene become pregnant at the

50-milligram dose and 20 percent do so at the 100-milligram dose. A smaller percentage of women may benefit from taking the drug for seven or eights days in a row. Overall, from 60 percent to 90 percent of women who take clomiphene will ovulate, and up to one half will become pregnant. In any one treatment cycle, from 12 percent to 25 percent of women who ovulate will conceive.

The side effects of clomiphene include hot flashes, mood swings, depression, headaches, pelvic pain, nausea, and breast tenderness. Visual symptoms such as blurring, halos, and streaks of light at night are more serious side effects. If significant side effects occur, the drug is discontinued immediately. About 10 percent of women who get pregnant with clomiphene have a multiple pregnancy, usually twins.

The antiestrogen effects of clomiphene also affect the quality of cervical mucus. Up to 15 percent of women may have dry cervical mucus. Some fertility specialists recommend adding a small amount of estrogen to increase cervical mucus, but there's no evidence that this significantly increases pregnancy rates.

Clomiphene can also be combined with the drug metformin to treat women with polycystic ovary syndrome (PCOS). Metformin is an oral drug used to manage diabetes, either alone or in combination with sulfonylureas or other agents. To identify whether an infertile woman who has PCOS will benefit from metformin, simple tests are performed to see whether she has insulin resistance. If she does, then metformin is prescribed. Over two or three weeks, she slowly builds up to the usual dose of 500 milligrams of metformin three times daily or 850 milligrams twice daily with meals. If she does not start ovulating regularly over the next six to eight weeks, then clomiphene treatment is initiated.

Women with PCOS typically have high blood levels of androgens. This may be due to too much output of dehydroepiandrosterone sulfate (DHEAS) from the adrenal glands. A woman with PCOS and high DHEAS levels may benefit from additional treatment with the steroid medication dexamethasone along with the clomiphene therapy. Dexamethasone reduces the secretion of adrenocorticotropic hormone from the pituitary, which in turn reduces the production of adrenal hormones.

Dr. Rosenwaks initially prescribes a low dose of 0.25 milligram of dexamethasone at night and may increase the dose as high as 0.5 milligram. Adding dexamethasone to clomiphene may help to induce ovulation in women with PCOS who have particularly high levels of androgens from the adrenal gland.

Human Menopausal Gonadotropins

When a woman doesn't respond to clomiphene, she may benefit from treatment with gonadotropins, either FSH alone or in combination with LH. These come in preparations containing equal amounts of bioactive FSH and LH with human menopausal gonadotropin (hMG, Pergonal, Repronex, Menopur), which are extracted from menopausal women's urine. Pergonal and hMG are usually injected into the muscle. Repronex and Menopur and two similar drugs, highly purified FSH (Fertinex, Bravelle) and newer, genetically engineered versions of FSH (Gonal-F, Follistim), can be administered under the skin by subcutaneous injection.

In contrast to clomiphene, gonadotropins induce ovulation by directly stimulating the ovaries. The FSH in the drug travels through the blood into the ovaries to stimulate the growth of follicles. And since it does not interfere with estrogen production, it does not disrupt cervical mucus production as clomiphene does. Recently, long-acting hybrid gonadotropin preparations requiring fewer injections have been introduced, but they are still being investigated.

A woman with hypogonadotropic hypogonadism who does not respond to clomiphene treatments usually does well with gonadotropin therapy. Dr. Rosenwaks starts her off on a dosage of 75 to 150 international units daily. He adjusts the dose based on ultrasound scans and estradiol levels. When one follicle has matured, he administers human chorionic gonadotropin (hCG) at a dose of 5,000 to 10,000 international units either intramuscularly or subcutaneously. The hCG acts like LH to stimulate the egg to mature fully and for the follicle to rupture and release the egg. It's usually administered the day after the last dose of hMG, and ovulation occurs about thirty-six to thirty-nine hours later.

Gonadotropin therapy has to be monitored carefully to avoid ovarian hyperstimulation syndrome, in which too many follicles are stimulated and the ovaries become enlarged. The syndrome can range from mild discomfort to severe illness, which may require hospitalization. That's why Dr. Rosenwaks uses the lowest effective dose, takes multiple ultrasound scans, and obtains frequent estradiol measurements after a woman begins gonadotropin therapy. If a woman starts to respond too much—her ovaries go from the size of golf balls to the size of grapefruits—he takes her off the drug and withholds the gonadotropins. He also advises the couple to avoid intercourse to prevent pregnancy in case she ovulates spontaneously. An inadvertent pregnancy can exacerbate the problem due to increasing hCG produced in a pregnancy. One of the newer ways to administer gonadotropins in women with PCOS is to start the medication at the lowest possible dose and increase the dose slowly over a period of two to three weeks. The aim is for the woman to develop a single follicle.

Another potential complication of the therapy is a multiple pregnancy, since gonadotropin stimulates follicle growth. The chances of a multiple pregnancy are directly related to the number of mature follicles that develop during gonadotropin therapy. About 20 percent of women who take gonadotropins have multiple pregnancies, most often twins.

Gonadotropin-Releasing Hormone

A woman who has weak hormonal signals from the hypothalamus to the pituitary and doesn't ovulate after taking clomiphene may be a candidate to take GnRH. This therapy is effective for those women with hypogonadotropic hypogonadism who have normal pituitary function; that is, their primary problem is an inadequate amount of GnRH secreted by the hypothalamus.

The GnRH is administered in pulses to mimic what happens naturally in the body. The woman receives 5-microgram doses into a vein (intravenously) every sixty to ninety minutes or 10-microgram doses subcutaneously every ninety minutes via a portable infusion pump worn on a belt around the waist. This treatment usually culminates with a single developed follicle and spontaneous ovulation. If spontaneous ovulation does not occur, Dr. Rosenwaks administers five thousand to ten thousand international units of hCG to induce ovulation and, rarely, follows with one thousand to two thousand international units every three days to support the luteal phase of her cycle. About 80 percent of women with hypogonadotropic hypogonadism will ovulate and roughly 25 percent will become pregnant in any given cycle of GnRH treatment.

GnRH has advantages over hMG: a negligible risk of hyperstimulation and fewer multiple pregnancies (only about 5 percent). The drug is more effective and more reliable when given through a vein, but this requires monitoring of the intravenous line. Having a catheter in a vein for up to three weeks at a time raises the risk of potentially dangerous infections and sepsis. Common side effects with delivery through the pump include pain, swelling and infection at the infusion site. Practically, this approach is more cumbersome than subcutaneous administration of gonadotropins and is rarely used.

Risk of Ovarian Cancer

Some earlier studies suggested that women treated with fertility hormones had an increased risk of ovarian cancer. Recent studies have not confirmed these risks. In fact, it appears that it is not the fertility drugs, but rather the duration of the infertility and a lack of use of birth control pills that may increase the risk of ovarian cancer. Generally, ovulation-inducing drugs are safe as long as they are used for appropriate indications, are monitored properly, and are not used excessively. Any drug or medical procedure, if used excessively or inappropriately, may have associated risks, and some of those risks may have not yet been identified.

Other Drugs Used for Fertility Treatments

Endometriosis

From one quarter to one third of infertile women have endometriosis. The disease develops when endometrial tissue from the inner lining of the uterus grows in other locations, typically around the ovaries, fallopian tubes, and other pelvic organs. But no one knows why some women develop endometriosis. The immune system is most likely involved, and some women may have a genetic predisposition toward the disease.

Many women with endometriosis have no symptoms at all, and the fertility specialist often makes the diagnosis incidentally during a laparoscopy for other problems. Some women with extensive endometriosis have little or no pain, but the typical symptoms include pelvic pain, painful bowel movements, back pain, abdominal bloating, and pain during intercourse.

The scars that form on the ovaries and fallopian tubes may impair a woman's fertility. A woman who has no physical damage from endometriosis may have impaired ovulation, a reduced response to hormonal stimulation of her ovaries, poor embryo quality, and faulty embryo implantation.

Medical treatment of endometriosis is used mainly to control symptoms and manage recurrences. The best method of suppressing endometriosis is with GnRH agonists leuprolide (Lupron), goserelin (Zoladex), or nafarelin (Synarel). These are synthetic versions of GnRH that are many times more potent than the natural hormone. They initially cause a greater release of pituitary hormones, but the long duration of action of GnRH agonists quickly depletes LH and FSH from the pituitary. This stops the production of estrogens and, as a result, inhibits the growth of endometriosis, which is dependent on estrogens.

The three versions of GnRH are administered in three different forms. Leuprolide is usually given as a once-a-month injection, goserelin as a monthly subcutaneous implant, and nafarelin as a twice-a-day nasal spray.

The side effects of GnRH agonists are similar to those of menopause, including hot flashes, vaginal dryness, headaches, depression, and decreased sex drive. The long-term use of these drugs can lead to osteoporosis. Once GnRH agonist treatment goes beyond six months, it is recommended that a woman add either pure progestin (5 mg of norethindrone) or a combination of low-dose estrogen (0.625 mg of conjugated equine estrogen) with a progestin to reduce the woman's loss of bone mineral density.

Another treatment option is a progestin, such as medroxyprogesterone, which can be prescribed in a 30-milligram daily pill. This is a less expensive therapy with fewer side effects, which include weight gain, fluid retention, breakthrough bleeding before or after menstruation, and depression.

Danocrine (danazol), a synthetic derivative of the steroid testosterone, used to be the drug of choice for endometriosis. Danocrine counteracts the effects of estrogen and induces a menopausal-like state. But in addition to menopausal side effects, this drug also produces masculinizing effects, such as growth of facial hair, acne, and a decrease in breast size, and therefore is no longer commonly used.

Uterine Fibroids

Dr. Rosenwaks may also use GnRH agonists to treat uterine fibroids. These benign tumors arise from the muscle cells of the uterus. About two thirds of women with uterine fibroids have no symptoms. When symptoms occur, a woman may feel abdominal discomfort and pressure from a growing fibroid. She may also complain of heavy menstruation and/or irregular uterine bleeding. GnRH agonist treatment is often a temporary measure to stop uterine bleeding.

Uterine fibroids are rarely the sole cause of infertility. The location of uterine fibroids may dictate whether they interfere with implantation or obstruct the fallopian tubes. Multiple fibroids, especially if they are large and are located near the cavity of the uterus, may cause recurrent miscarriages. The most effective treatment for fibroids is to remove them surgically. When large, fibroids may be shrunk with GnRH agonist treatments before surgery. Since GnRH agonists suppress estrogen secretion, and fibroids need estrogen to grow, this therapy is very effective in reducing the size of large fibroids. This pretreatment may reduce blood loss during subsequent surgery to remove the remaining fibroids and can also reduce the need for blood transfusion during the surgery. Fibroids may be removed by an abdominal approach (laparotomy), by a laparoscopy or, if they are in the uterine cavity, by hysteroscopy.

Pituitary Tumors

Drug therapy is the mainstay of treatment for prolactin-secreting pituitary tumors. The drug bromocriptine mesylate (Parlodel) is highly effective in reducing prolactin levels and inducing regression of tumors.

By suppressing production of prolactin from the pituitary, bromocriptine restores the normal flow of hormones to the ovaries. It is particularly helpful for women who have high blood levels of prolactin and do not menstruate or ovulate. Those women with hypogonadotropic hypogonadism whose disease is due to high prolactin levels respond well to the drug.

Dr. Rosenwaks commonly prescribes 2.5 milligrams of bromocriptine orally or vaginally twice daily. He monitors prolactin blood levels to confirm that they have returned to normal, and adjusts the drug dosage if necessary. A woman's menstrual function is generally restored within six months, and about 70 percent of women become pregnant after bromocriptine therapy.

The side effects of bromocriptine include dizziness, nausea, low blood pressure, and nasal congestion. These can be minimized by starting at a low dose of the drug at bedtime and gradually increasing the dose.

For the past several years a long-acting medication called cabergoline

(Dostinex) has also been successfully used to treat hyperprolactinemia. The dose is usually 0.5 milligram twice per week.

Surgical Treatments

Abnormalities of the fallopian tubes and uterus are responsible for a significant portion of female infertility. Tubal adhesions, tubal obstruction, and malformation of the reproductive tract are common anatomical problems associated with infertility. In rare cases, strategically placed cervical or uterine polyps, if large, may also cause fertility problems. Simple outpatient procedures through a laparoscope or hysteroscope, as well as delicate operations using microsurgery, can correct these problems and help couples conceive.

Laparoscopic Surgery

Using contemporary surgical instruments and techniques, laparoscopic surgery can be used to free adhesions (scars) due to previous pelvic inflammatory disease (PID), treat endometriosis, or remove ovarian cysts and even ectopic (tubal or ovarian) pregnancies. These procedures can be performed on a single-day outpatient basis. Any anatomic conditions diagnosed during laparoscopy can often be treated immediately. Even more sophisticated operations, such as removing uterine fibroids or microsurgical repair of the fallopian tubes, can be performed through the laparoscope. In fact, properly trained fertility specialists can use robotic techniques through the laparoscope to perform the most sophisticated pelvic corrective procedures with one-day outpatient surgery. Our hospital and reproductive surgeons are trained in all these contemporary approaches.

Laparoscopic surgery is an effective approach for excising endometriosis and for removing any associated adhesions. Excision of endometriomas is the preferred method of treating ovarian endometriosis, although, on occasion, vaporization of deep-seated endometrioma is the only way to treat the disease completely. It is important to send tissue to the pathology lab for analysis to confirm the diagnosis and to insure that no malignant tissue exists within it.

Women with mild to moderate endometriosis are more likely to become pregnant after laparoscopic surgery than after medical therapy. In advanced endometriosis, surgery is definitely the treatment of choice because large endometrial cysts do not respond well to medical therapy.

An ectopic pregnancy usually indicates that a woman has some sort of damage to her fallopian tubes. Dr. Rosenwaks usually uses conservative laparoscopic surgery to make an incision in the fallopian tube to remove the ectopic pregnancy or may remove the section of the tube containing the ectopic pregnancy. When the tube is damaged and swollen, it may be preferable to remove it rather than try to save it.

In general, most corrective pelvic surgery can be performed through the laparoscope. If this is not possible, then open surgery through a regular abdominal surgical incision may be necessary.

The risks of laparoscopic surgery are the same as any operation, including bleeding, infection, and complications from the anesthesia. In addition, the surgery may injure the intestines or urinary tract, or cause internal bleeding, which requires immediate open surgery to control the bleeding.

The typical symptoms following a laparoscopy include shoulder, chest, and upper abdominal pain from the carbon dioxide gas left in the woman's abdominal cavity. She may feel bloated and have some tenderness around the small incisions, which usually improves after a few days.

Surgery for Tubal Disease

Tubal disease is responsible for a significant proportion of female infertility. Any anatomic distortion that interferes with the fallopian tube's ability to pick up or move the egg can cause infertility. As mentioned above, tubal obstruction can occur at the far end (distal part) of the fallopian tube or near the uterine end. Sometimes the tubes are encased in filmy adhesions (scars) that do not allow the tubes to move properly or prevent the tube from picking up the egg. Successful repair of fallopian tube disease is very much dependent on the severity and type of abnormality.

In mild cases releasing the filmy adhesions surrounding the tubes and ovaries can be performed through the laparoscope. Sometimes adhesions surround the fingerlike opening (fimbria) at the far end of the tube and partially block the tube. If this is the case, Dr. Rosenwaks cuts and removes the band of adhesions surrounding the tube. About 45 percent of women will become pregnant within two years after this procedure.

Surgery to repair blocked tubes at the far end can be done through a laparoscope or by open surgery with similar success rates. The most important factor is the extent of damage to the tubes. There's no benefit in using lasers to open up the tubes in terms of pregnancy rates. Almost three quarters of women with mild disease will conceive after surgery. Those with moderate to severe disease have a worse prognosis—less than 30 percent will conceive after surgery.

The risk of ectopic pregnancy also relates to the extent of the disease. Women with mild disease who have surgery to reconstruct their tubes have between a 5 percent and a 10 percent risk of an ectopic pregnancy. As the severity of the disease worsens, the chance of ectopic pregnancy increases.

Whenever possible, Dr. Rosenwaks attempts to treat tubal problems using laparoscopic surgery, which has the benefits of a shorter recovery and hospital stay, lower risk of new adhesions forming, and less postoperative pain.

In some instances fallopian tubes are blocked at the end near the uterus. This can be visualized during a hysterosalpingogram when the fertility specialist observes that no dye has reached the middle or far end of the tube. However, the injection of dye into the tube may send it into spasm, and it closes temporarily. If the tubes cannot be visualized on a hysterosalpingogram, then a hysteroscope can be used to insert a guide wire into the near end of the tube. Most often, a mucus plug is blocking this part of the tube, and this simple procedure relieves the obstruction, resulting in a pregnancy rate of 40 percent within one year.

If this doesn't work, the next step is surgical correction of the blocked portion of the tube. Pregnancy success rates depend on the extent of damage at the time of surgery, with about 50 percent of women becoming pregnant.

Dr. Rosenwaks often recommends IVF rather than surgery when the damage to the woman's fallopian tubes is severe, particularly if the far end of the tube is totally blocked, or when previous surgical attempts have failed. Fluid leaking from the far end of the tube into the uterus can prevent the embryo from implanting. Also, although there is no age cutoff for surgery, women age thirty-seven and older have a significantly lower chance of success with tubal surgery, and he usually encourages the couple to proceed with IVF as soon as possible. Often, a single cycle of IVF offers the same or better chance of conception than undergoing tubal surgery and waiting for one year.

Sterilization Reversal

Sterilization procedures that destroy the least amount of the fallopian tubes have the highest success rates after reversal. Reversal after a surgical clip or ring was used results in a chance of better than 80 percent for pregnancy after surgical repair. Tubes that were cut by heat or electrical current yield much lower success rates and may even be irreversible if significant segments of the tubes were destroyed. If less than 4 centimeters of each tube is available, the chance of a successful reversal is poor.

Other factors that limit the success of a reversal include a large discrepancy in the diameter of the two segments to be connected, the period of time elapsing between procedures, and whether the woman is obese. To obtain the best results, the fertility specialist can utilize either an open abdominal incision under general anesthesia or a laparoscopic incision using a robotic technique. In both instances, microsurgical techniques are used to reconnect the tubes using needles as thin as human hair and even thinner thread. The laparoscopic approach is performed as a one-day procedure; the abdominal approach requires a three-to-five-day hospital stay.

Surgery for Uterine Fibroids

The size, shape, and location of uterine fibroids determine whether they should be removed through the laparoscope or through the abdomen in open surgery.

The easiest fibroids to remove through the laparoscope are attached to the outside of the uterus by a stalk. Many fibroids close to the outer surface of the uterus can also be removed laparoscopically. Those that are found deep within the uterine wall are the most difficult to remove with the laparoscope. Dr. Rosenwaks usually removes deep or multiple fibroids through an abdominal incision and open surgery.

Laparoscopic and abdominal surgery to remove uterine fibroids both require general anesthesia and a hospital stay of about two days. The recovery from laparoscopic surgery takes about four weeks, with an additional two weeks for abdominal surgery.

Hysteroscopic Surgery

A hysteroscope can be used both to diagnose and to treat abnormalities of the uterine cavity. Because the hysteroscope goes through the cervix, the doctor does not need to make any incisions. Procedures using the hysteroscope are done as outpatient surgery under local or general anesthesia.

The hysteroscope is a highly efficient instrument for surgical removal and correction of lesions in the uterine cavity. These include small fibroids (also called submucosal myomas) immediately under the lining of the uterus, a fibrous band that distorts the cavity and may cause miscarriages (called a uterine septum), polyps, and adhesions caused by scarring of the endometrial cavity (Asherman syndrome). Scar tissue within the uterus is often the result of an abortion, infection following a dilation and curettage after miscarriage, or even a postcesarean or delivery-associated infection. The risks of hysteroscopic surgery include bleeding, infection, uterine perforation, and anesthesia-related complications.

Intrauterine Insemination

If a man's sperm count is low or his sperm motility is poor, or antisperm antibodies factor into a couple's failure to conceive, then Dr. Rosenwaks may suggest they try ovulation induction plus intrauterine insemination (IUI). If an extensive workup of both partners fails to find any reasons for their infertility—what's called unexplained infertility—they are also good candidates for this procedure.

The concept is simple: induce ovulation of more than one egg using hormone treatments and then, just after ovulation, place all of the washed moving sperm into the uterus to ease their passage to the eggs.

Ovulation induction can be performed using standard doses of clomiphene citrate from day 3 to day 7 or day 5 to day 9 of the menstrual cycle. On day 10 to day 11 of the cycle, careful monitoring for the LH surge is begun. The IUI is performed twenty-four to twenty-six hours after the LH surge is detected. If no LH surge is detected by day 14 to 15 and a dominant preovulatory follicle is observed on ultrasound, hCG can be administered to induce ovulation.

Once the timing of the IUI is set, the man collects a sperm sample either at home or in Dr. Rosenwaks's office. His sperm are then processed using a "swim–up" technique. The semen is placed at the bottom of a gradient gel, and the sperm compete against each other to swim to the top of the gel. The winners of the race are skimmed off the top. The best swimmers usually also have better sperm shape. This process provides better-quality sperm than the simple "wash" used by many labs, and also eliminates white blood cells and debris, which are not good for sperm. These sperm are drawn up into a flexible plastic catheter. Dr. Rosenwaks gently inserts the catheter through the cervix into the woman's uterus and deposits the sperm. He also encourages the couple to have intercourse on the day of and the day after the insemination to enhance the chances of pregnancy.

The sperm washing takes from thirty to sixty minutes, and the IUI itself takes several minutes. After the insemination, the woman lies on her back for about ten minutes. Then she gets up and can resume her normal activities.

Three to five days after the IUI, progesterone levels are checked. If they are low, supplements are given to support the luteal phase of the cycle. She either uses a vaginal suppository containing 200 milligrams of progesterone at bedtime or twice daily or applies a crystalized (micronized) version of the drug vaginally three times a day for seven weeks.

If the couple doesn't conceive during the first cycle, they try again for three to six cycles. Within six months, 30 percent to 50 percent of couples with unexplained infertility will conceive, although pregnancy rates diminish with advancing age. Overall, 10 percent to 20 percent of couples will conceive in any one IUI cycle.

For women who don't respond to initial doses of clomiphene, Dr. Rosenwaks may extend the duration of clomiphene for a few more days or may change to more powerful gonadotropins, either combinations of FSH and LH or pure FSH, to stimulate the ovaries. He carefully monitors the development of follicles and blood levels of estradiol to reduce the risk of ovarian hyperstimulation.

If a woman doesn't develop any mature follicles after taking ovulation-inducing drugs, the IUI is canceled. On the other hand, if she develops four or more mature follicles and has high estradiol levels, the IUI could be canceled because of the increased risk of multiple pregnancies. In this situation, Dr. Rosenwaks may encourage the couple to convert to an IVF cycle. Dr. Rosenwaks's research shows that couples can safely switch from IUI to a standard IVF attempt. Conversely, a couple destined for IVF in which the woman has healthy fallopian tubes can switch to an IUI if follicle development and egg yield are likely to be low.

Repeated Pregnancy Loss

Miscarriages occur more often than people realize. In women younger than age thirty-four, approximately 10 percent of all pregnancies result in miscarriages, while in women who are forty-five or older, more than 50 percent to 60 percent of pregnancies are lost. When a woman has had three or more consecutive miscarriages, there is a reasonable likelihood that there is a medical or genetic cause for her miscarriages. In fact, it is recommended that all couples who have more than two miscarriages undergo a recurrent pregnancy loss evaluation. Miscarriages can be caused by medical conditions, endocrine or anatomic problems, as well as by genetic defects or environmental factors.

Hormonal disorders related to thyroid disease, poorly controlled diabetes, malnutrition, or even pituitary tumors may lead to pregnancy loss. Specific problems with progesterone production after ovulation—the so-called luteal phase defect—can lead to implantation problems and early miscarriages. The majority of miscarriages, more than 60 percent to 70 percent, are caused by chromosomal abnormalities, due to either too few or too many chromosomes in the early embryo. Most commonly this is the result of maternal aging and egg abnormalities. In less than 10 percent of miscarriages the underlying cause is a chromosomal abnormality inherited from either the father or mother; most chromosomal abnormalities are the result of too few or too many chromosomes in the mother's egg at fertilization.

When there is a problem in one of the parents, preimplantation genetic diagnosis or screening (PGD/PGS) in combination with IVF can screen for these abnormalities in the embryo. This can generally be used successfully when the parents have a chromosomal abnormality that causes the embryo to inherit too many or too few chromosomes. In PGD/PGS, a single cell is removed from the early embryo to assess whether it's normal. Transferring only the "normal" embryos can reduce the chance for a miscarriage.

Approximately 15 percent of women with recurrent miscarriages have an anatomic defect. This may be a septum of the uterus, scarring in the uterine cavity, or even a one-sided (unicornuate) uterus. Occasionally a fibroid distorts the implantation bed in the uterus or a woman has a uterine defect that can lead to miscarriages. Such anatomic defects can be corrected by hysteroscopy.

Other important causes of repeated miscarriage include autoimmune diseases, the presence of antiphospholipid antibodies, or problems with blood clotting. Treatment of these specific disorders may require special therapy with blood thinners, cortisone-like drugs, and baby aspirin. It is important to remember that in many instances doctors cannot find an obvious reason for the miscarriages and that 60 percent of these women become pregnant without treatment.

In the Future

Many of the present treatments for infertility require injections of hormones and invasive surgical procedures. In the future, new methods of drug delivery may make needles obsolete. Similarly, new hormones may be discovered that may substitute for present therapies.

Kisspeptin Kick-Starts LH and FSH

A hormone that plays a crucial role in the onset of puberty may also become a fertility treatment that kick-starts the female reproductive system. British researchers conducted a small study of infertile women who had stopped ovulating due to an imbalance in the sex hormones LH and FSH. Those women who received kisspeptin injections showed marked increases in their blood levels of LH and FSH compared to the women who received placebo injections.

The drug directly stimulates the release of GnRH, which then stimulates LH and FSH production in the pituitary. The researchers believe kisspeptin can be developed into a less risky hormone than combinations of FSH and LH or pure FSH, which often stimulate the ovaries to produce more than one egg. More eggs mean a higher risk of multiple pregnancies.

Kisspeptin is far from a panacea, and much more research in larger groups of infertile women is necessary. But if future studies pan out, then the 10 percent of infertile women with hormonal imbalances may have another option for ovulation induction.

Fertility Patch Stimulates Hormone Production

You've heard of nicotine patches to help smokers quit, as well as skin patches to relieve pain or to prevent seasickness. Infertile women may be able to use a skin patch to receive pulses of GnRH in the same way the body delivers the hormone.

A study is under way to test the safety and effectiveness of a new delivery method of GnRH for women who are trying to get pregnant. The Lutre-patch delivers a GnRH dose every ninety minutes by an electrical impulse that drives the hormone across the skin and into the body. Unlike GnRH injections, which may overstimulate egg production, the patch delivers the hormone like the brain does naturally. This reduces the risk of multiple eggs being released, which would reduce the chance of multiple pregnancies.

The patch is now going through clinical trials at thirty-five fertility clin-ics across the country and likely won't hit the market for several years.

• • • • • • •

Infertility treatments are usually most effective within the first three to six cycles. After that, if a couple has not conceived, we generally counsel cou-ples to consider more aggressive therapy. In many cases, that means using assisted reproductive technologies and treatments such as IVF, which is the subject of the next chapter.

Take-Home Messages

- Hormone treatments can normalize the flow of hormones in your body or help time the release of an egg to optimize fertilization.
- Medications can control the symptoms of endometriosis and help manage recurrences. Surgery is the best way to remove endometriomas completely.
- Surgery through a laparoscope can free scar tissue from pelvic inflammatory disease, treat endometriosis, or remove an ectopic pregnancy or ovarian cysts. Surgery is the most effective treatment for endometriosis.
- A blockage in the fallopian tubes is one of the most common causes of female infertility.

- Surgery through a hysteroscope is an efficient method of removing certain tissues from the uterus and treating intrauterine problems.
- Intrauterine insemination may be a good fertility option if the man has a low sperm count or you have a diagnosis of unexplained infertility.
- If you have had two or more miscarriages, both you and your partner need a thorough evaluation to investigate the cause.

Part III

Advanced Technologies and Treatments

Ten

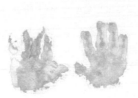

Am I a Candidate for IVF?

When to Do In Vitro Fertilization

. . . .

When George, an attorney, turned thirty, a routine physical showed he had low hormone levels. He consulted a urologist, who found George also had a low sperm count. "That explained why I couldn't get pregnant," says his wife Martha, a thirty-year-old meeting planner. They went to see Dr. Goldstein, who confirmed George's problem and recommended they try intrauterine insemination (IUI). Two IUI cycles failed, so they scheduled an in vitro fertilization (IVF) cycle with Dr. Rosenwaks. "He told us our chances were good, and he was right. I got pregnant the first time," says Martha. Their daughter Suzanne is now four years old.

. . . .

Almost a quarter of a million babies are born each year through assisted reproductive technology (ART) procedures, and nearly 4 million babies worldwide have been born using a remarkable technique that combines sperm and eggs outside the body, known as IVF. This ART procedure retrieves multiple eggs and mixes them with sperm in the laboratory, and the embryos that grow in a special culture medium are then transplanted into the uterus.

More than 115,000 IVF treatment cycles are performed in the United States each year, and this figure continues to grow at a steady pace. An IVF cycle costs between $10,000 and $15,000, and on average, a woman requires more than one cycle to achieve a pregnancy. For each cycle, a woman undergoes hormone injections to stimulate her ovaries, the eggs are removed and fertilized outside the body, and the resulting embryos are then transferred back into the uterus with the hope that an implantation will occur several days later.

About half of all women under age thirty-five, 40 percent of all women who are thirty-five and thirty-six, and one third of women who are thirty-seven through forty will have a baby after a single IVF transfer at Weill Cornell.

Candidates for IVF

Couples who require IVF treatment fall into many categories. No matter what the cause of their infertility, if conventional treatment has not resulted in a pregnancy, they become candidates for IVF.

Candidates for IVF include couples with tubal-factor infertility; couples where the male partner has severely compromised semen parameters (decreased sperm density, motility, and/or morphology); when the man has no sperm in the ejaculate, due to either obstruction or poor or no sperm production; women of advanced maternal age and diminished ovarian reserve; women with untreatable endometriosis; couples with unexplained infertility or antisperm antibodies; and even couples who carry genetic abnormalities and do not want to pass these on to their children.

IVF was originally devised to bypass the need for a healthy fallopian tube, where the sperm and egg normally meet for fertilization. Currently, when a woman has obstructed tubes or scarring around her fallopian tubes, her options are surgery or IVF. If a woman is older than thirty-five or if she has had unsuccessful tubal surgery, Dr. Rosenwaks generally recommends IVF as the best treatment. However, a sterilization reversal using microsurgery to reconnect the fallopian tubes may be the best choice for a woman under age thirty-five who has had a sterilization procedure, has a normal ovarian reserve, wishes to have more than one child, and has an adequate amount of tube left to repair. For all other women with tubal infertility, IVF may be a better option, because it doesn't require general anesthesia or major surgery.

The severity of a man's infertility dictates the best treatment. If he has at least 5 million active sperm, Dr. Rosenwaks generally recommends intrauterine insemination (IUI), either in a natural cycle or with ovarian stimulation (superovulation) of his female partner. If the couple doesn't achieve a pregnancy with IUI or the man has less than 500,000 active sperm, then Dr. Rosenwaks recommends IVF with intracytoplasmic sperm injection (ICSI).

Sperm Density Necessary for Achieving Pregnancy

Reproductive Method	Number of Sperm
Natural	≥ 20 million
IUI	≥ 2–5 million
IVF	≥ 500,000
ICSI	≥ 1

≥ = greater than or equal to

As noted above, a woman's age as well as her ovarian reserve, which reflects the biologic age of her ovaries, is critical to determining her fertility potential. To get a sense of a woman's ovarian reserve, Dr. Rosenwaks measures her blood levels of follicle-stimulating hormone (FSH), estradiol, and anti-Müllerian hormone (AMH) on day 3 of her cycle. A high FSH level indicates a woman has a diminishing ovarian reserve and suggests she may need more aggressive treatment. AMH levels can be used to confirm the diagnosis; low levels denote poor ovarian reserve. A clomiphene challenge test can help confirm a diminished ovarian reserve. No test result should absolutely eliminate or preclude treatment. Dr. Rosenwaks encourages women of any age with diminishing ovarian reserve as well as women age thirty-six and older to have an IVF procedure sooner rather than later.

When endometriosis does not respond to medical or surgical treatments or a woman is age thirty-five or older, then IVF should be the couple's treatment of choice.

Couples with unexplained infertility who do not get pregnant during several cycles of superovulation plus IUI are often quite successful with an IVF procedure. The IVF procedure allows Dr. Rosenwaks to evaluate sperm and egg interaction directly and also to evaluate the quality of the embryos. In fact, couples with unexplained infertility have higher pregnancy rates with IVF than couples in which the woman has a tubal problem.

Antisperm antibodies can be managed with IUI, IVF, or ICSI. IUI plus superovulation is the least expensive option but does not work as well as

IVF or ICSI. IUI may be successful when levels of antisperm antibodies are low. Dr. Rosenwaks recommends IVF when the woman has antisperm antibodies in her blood or her cervix or when a man has more than 50 percent of his sperm bound with antibodies. Couples with antisperm antibodies who undergo IVF have the same success rate as those without antibodies. ICSI is the most expensive of these procedures, but it has the highest success rate because the direct injection of sperm into the egg completely bypasses any antibodies either in the female or male.

Fertility specialists now have the ability to examine embryos in the laboratory before they are implanted. This has expanded the uses of IVF technology to help avoid the transmission of some genetic disorders. Preimplantation genetic diagnosis (PGD) can identify chromosomal abnormalities related to a woman's advancing age from a single cell removed from a three-day-old embryo, as well as detect specific genetic defects such as cystic fibrosis and sickle cell anemia.

The IVF Procedure

Before a couple has an IVF procedure at Weill Cornell, Dr. Rosenwaks makes sure they have undergone a thorough fertility evaluation. He documents that the woman's uterus is normal with a hysterosalpingogram or ultrasound scan. The man has a semen analysis to determine whether standard IVF or ICSI would be the best procedure. It's important for the man to have two to three sperm specimens frozen before IVF if he anticipates having difficulty producing a specimen on demand or if he has a very low sperm count. Generally, Dr. Rosenwaks asks the man to take an oral antibiotic during the first portion of an IVF cycle. This reduces the possibility of having bacteria in the sperm sample produced at the time of egg retrieval and reduces possible problems with fertilization and embryo development.

To ensure the embryo transfer goes smoothly, Dr. Rosenwaks puts the woman through a mock (or trial) embryo transfer in a pre-IVF cycle. This involves passing an empty catheter through the cervix into the uterus to verify that a real embryo transfer can be done easily and to measure the distance to the top of the woman's uterine cavity.

To develop more than one follicle, he uses various fertility drugs, a process known as controlled ovarian hyperstimulation. Several hormone preparations are available, including recombinant FSH for delivery under the skin (subcutaneously) or human menopausal gonadotropin (hMG), which contains a combination of FSH and LH and can be delivered either under the skin or into a muscle by injection. The woman takes these drugs for one or two weeks.

Most often, the woman starts daily hormone injections on cycle days 2 or 3 of her menstrual cycle. The dosage is tailored according to the woman's individual needs, considering her age, ovarian reserve—especially the number of small follicles in her ovaries (antral follicle counts)—weight, body mass index, and, when available, her response to previous stimulation cycles. Dr. Rosenwaks adjusts the dosage depending on her ovaries' response and the size of the follicles as measured by ultrasound. Usually he uses a step-down approach that reduces the drug dosage typically after two to four days of stimulation, once the follicles begin to enlarge and develop. This reduces the total amounts of drug delivered and reduces the risk of overstimulation as well as the cost of the IVF stimulation drugs.

To prevent the woman from ovulating before her eggs are retrieved, he may administer a gonadotropin-releasing hormone (GnRH) agonist, depending on the particular needs of the woman. GnRH agonists have both positive and negative effects on the pituitary gland. For the first few days of treatment, they stimulate the pituitary to release FSH and LH. After one week, they desensitize the pituitary to inhibit FSH and LH. This seemingly contradictory effect can be used to the patient's advantage. If total suppression is required, patients must take the medication for ten to fourteen days before FSH and LH are administered. When a stimulatory effect is desired, patients can begin GnRH agonist treatment along with gonadotropins, allowing their own FSH and LH to complement the injected FSH and LH.

Alternatively, he may administer a faster-acting medicine, similar to GnRH agonists, called a GnRH antagonist, either cetrorelix acetate (Cetrotide) or ganirelix acetate (Antagon). GnRH antagonists prevent the release of gonadotropins by the pituitary immediately after administration. They lower the levels of FSH and LH within four to eight hours, much more quickly than GnRH agonists.

Egg Retrieval and Embryo Transfer

When IVF was first introduced, eggs were retrieved for IVF via the laparoscope, but follicles deep inside the ovaries were often missed. Nowadays, eggs are retrieved through the vagina under ultrasound guidance. No general anesthesia is usually needed since an intravenous sedative acts rapidly and effectively. A needle is inserted into each follicle to aspirate the fluid, which is collected in a tube, and the tube is transferred to a laboratory next door to the operating room to identify the eggs.

Once the eggs reach the laboratory, they are placed in a special culture medium. The man's semen, which is usually collected just before the eggs are recovered, is washed, and the best sperm are separated out. Each egg is inseminated with fifty thousand to one hundred thousand moving sperm. If the man has severely low sperm quality, then Dr. Rosenwaks recommends an ICSI procedure for insemination.

The eggs and sperm are incubated for twelve to eighteen hours. The next day, the eggs are examined to see which ones are fertilized. The fertilized eggs remain in a culture medium for up to three to five days. An embryologist checks their progress and quality every twenty-four hours.

Three days after the egg retrieval, when the eggs have divided three times into a six- or eight-cell embryo, the embryos are placed into the uterus. If several embryos are available, Dr. Rosenwaks may delay the transfer until the fifth day, when the embryos have become blastocysts, so he can select the best embryos. Blastocyst transfers are generally used when there are more than eight embryos available, especially in women younger than thirty-six.

The embryo transfer is a simple ten-minute outpatient procedure that does not usually require anesthesia. Dr. Rosenwaks threads a soft, pliable catheter through the cervix into the uterus and deposits the embryos. The catheter contains a small amount of culture medium as well as the embryos. The woman rests for about thirty minutes and then goes home. She can resume normal activities on the following day. Implantation usually occurs seven to nine days after the eggs were collected.

The number of embryos transferred depends on the woman's age, her fertility history, and the embryo quality. Usually one to three embryos are transferred. However, with drugs stimulating the ovary to produce more follicles, it's not unusual to collect ten or more eggs, particularly in a young woman. The additional blastocysts that develop are frozen and preserved for possible future use.

Some women do not secrete enough progesterone after an IVF procedure, especially when secretion has been suppressed with a GnRH agonist during stimulation. To overcome this problem, Dr. Rosenwaks routinely supports the luteal phase of the menstrual cycle (the two weeks following the egg retrieval) with progesterone and occasionally with human chorionic gonadotropin (hCG), a hormone that stimulates the corpus luteum to secrete progesterone. He starts progesterone treatment one day after the egg retrieval with injections, vaginal suppositories, or capsules. He measures blood levels of progesterone and estradiol at ten, twelve, and fourteen days after the retrieval to make sure hormone levels are adequate to support the pregnancy. Some fertility clinics give small doses of hCG to increase the corpus luteum's production of progesterone, but this may increase the risk of ovarian hyperstimulation syndrome (OHSS).

The Risks of IVF

A carefully performed, ultrasound-guided vaginal IVF procedure is exceedingly safe. Even so, complications may develop. Some of the common side effects of stimulating the ovaries include tiredness, breast tenderness, pelvic pain, and mood swings. The most serious potential complication is overstimulation of the ovaries in response to hormone treatments, leading to OHSS. Careful cycle monitoring with dose adjustments reduces and virtually eliminates the risks of this syndrome. If it occurs, a woman can develop pain, weight gain, markedly enlarged ovaries, a significant increase in fluid in the pelvic area, abdominal swelling, and respiratory and kidney problems. In rare cases, OHSS has even been fatal.

The key is to prevent OHSS by tailoring the ovulation stimulation protocol for women at increased risk of overstimulation, which includes young women, those with polycystic ovary syndrome (PCOS), and those who have a history of OHSS. Historically, the most effective protocol for these women used low gonadotropin doses after the women's ovarian cycle was suppressed with oral contraceptives for twenty-eight days. Overlapping GnRH agonists were administered for the last seven days. In Dr. Rosenwaks's experience, this so-called "dual suppression" therapy was the most effective way to treat an abnormally high response to ovulation induction and allowed him to retrieve an optimum number of mature eggs. More recently, a protocol using oral contraceptives for twenty-one days without GnRH agonists has also been shown to be effective. This protocol requires ovulation suppression with GnRH antagonists at the end of the stimulation phase. This also gives Dr. Rosenwaks the option of triggering ovulation with a GnRH agonist.

Some women unexpectedly develop an abnormally high response to even modest amounts of stimulation drugs. Dr. Rosenwaks may simply cancel the cycle by stopping the ovulation-inducing drugs and withholding hCG, which eliminates the risk of OHSS. If the risk of OHSS is moderate, he may administer a reduced dose of hCG, retrieve the eggs, fertilize them, and freeze all of the embryos for transfer in a future IVF cycle.

Another alternative to just canceling the cycle is called "coasting." The doctor withholds ovulation drugs for one or more days while continuing pituitary suppression with a GnRH agonist. Within a few days, when the woman's estradiol levels drop to a safe level, he administers a reduced dose of hCG and continues the cycle. Fewer eggs are collected in "coasted" cycles, but pregnancy rates are still high. Usually, "coasting" avoids the need to freeze the embryos and postpone the actual embryo transfer. Because there's still a moderate risk of OHSS, Dr. Rosenwaks carefully monitors "coasted" cycles to determine whether it's safe to transfer embryos.

As more and more cycles of ovarian stimulation are performed with a GnRH antagonist to avoid LH surges, an innovative approach for avoiding OHSS has been the triggering of a short-lived LH surge with a GnRH agonist. A concentrated amount (bolus) of a GnRH agonist can overwhelm the pituitary inhibition of the antagonist, resulting in a normal LH surge. This avoids exposing the ovaries to the much longer stimulatory actions of hCG (the usual ovulatory trigger during ovulation induction). Early experience suggests that this may become the most effective method of avoiding OHSS.

Couples using IVF may also have a higher risk of preeclampsia, stillbirths, low-birth-weight babies, or babies that are small for gestational age. However, research has shown that IVF does not increase the risk of developmental disorders in these children as they grow up. In fact, one small University of Auckland study found IVF kids may grow taller and have a healthier metabolism than other children in their age group!

The embryo transfer may cause some cramping, discomfort, and possibly a small amount of bleeding. Infection is a possible result of the catheter insertion and may require antibiotic treatment.

Multiple Pregnancies

From its early beginnings, IVF success relied on the transfer of multiple embryos to overcome the relatively low embryo implantation rates. More recently, with improvements in technology and implantation efficiency, we have witnessed the emergence of a new problem, namely, the relatively high proportion of multiple pregnancies. Multiple pregnancies, especially high-order multiples, are associated with increased risks of premature delivery and increased medical complications for both mother and babies.

Publicity and media attention about several quintuplet pregnancies and even an octuplet pregnancy have placed intense scrutiny on fertility clinics to limit the number of embryos transferred and therefore reduce the chances of multiple pregnancies. With multiple pregnancies, there is a much higher rate of fetal loss and the risk of prematurity is exceedingly high. When very premature babies do survive, they are at risk for a host of medical complications, including respiratory problems, heart troubles, gastrointestinal problems, and a greater risk of infections. Preemies may have problems with nerve and brain development that may not be obvious until years later.

All multiple pregnancies increase the mother's risk of having hypertension (high blood pressure), gestational diabetes, toxemia, and other medical complications of pregnancy. Some risks may be life-threatening.

The goal of IVF treatments at Weill Cornell is for couples to have one healthy baby at a time. At Weill Cornell, we have steadily decreased the number of embryos we transfer, particularly in young women who are likely to have high embryo implantation rates. Whereas twenty years ago we might have transferred three or four embryos, today we prefer to transfer just one or two embryos.

One way the Weill Cornell IVF team limits multiple pregnancies is to select the healthiest embryos to transfer. When he retrieves many eggs, Dr. Rosenwaks allows the fertilized eggs to develop for five days, two more than usual, into the blastocyst stage. By virtue of developing to the blastocyst stage, an embryo has declared itself to be healthier. Blastocysts have a higher implantation rate than embryos that have been cultured for only three days. Transferring one or two blastocysts reduces the risk of high-order multiple pregnancies without compromising pregnancy rates. The only way to avoid multiple pregnancies is to transfer a single embryo.

Early Embryos

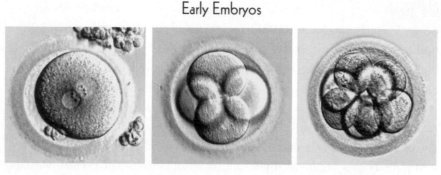

Day 1   Day 2   Day 3

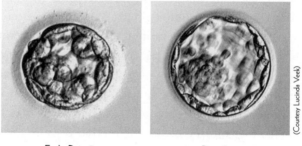

Early Day 5   Day 5

(Courtesy Lucinda Veek)

The American Society for Reproductive Medicine (ASRM) now recommends that women younger than thirty-five with a good prognosis should have just one or two embryos transferred. Women under age thirty-five make up about 40 percent of all IVF cycles. The ASRM guidelines recommend that women aged thirty-five to thirty-seven should have no more than three embryos or two blastocysts transferred. In women aged thirty-eight and older, who have a higher incidence of embryos with chromosomal defects, four embryos or three blastocysts (age thirty-eight to forty) or five embryos or three blastocysts (age forty and older) are recommended. When deciding on the number of embryos to be transferred, the number of failed cycles a woman has had, as well as the appearance and quality of transplanted embryos, has to be taken into consideration.

There is evidence that fertility clinics are reducing the number of multiple births and still maintaining high pregnancy rates. The database from the Society for Assisted Reproductive Technology (SART), one of the subspecialty societies of the ASRM, shows several important trends in 2007: the percentage of live births of triplets or more was below 2 percent, down from more than 6 percent in 2003, the average number of embryos transferred declined, and the percentages of cycles utilizing single embryo transfer was up.

Single-Embryo Transfer

An obvious way to reduce the risk of multiple pregnancies is to transfer a single embryo, although identical twins can occur under these circumstances if an embryo splits. Even more rarely, a single embryo can result in identical triplets. Many young women elect to have single-embryo transfer, especially in their first IVF attempt.

The main obstacle to single-embryo transfer is its lower success rate. To overcome that, some fertility specialists ask women to agree to two cycles, first transferring one fresh embryo while freezing others. If the first transfer fails, then a single frozen embryo is thawed and transferred. This approach yields similar success rates as transferring two embryos at once and drastically reduces the chances of twin pregnancies.

Another obstacle is not medical but the lack of insurance coverage. Many American couples lack insurance for IVF. At an average cost of about $12,500 a cycle, the costs of more than one IVF cycle can quickly add up. Some insurance companies will pay for only two IVF cycles, so couples opt to transfer multiple embryos at a time because they think that this is their only chance to complete their family. Studies show that couples with full insurance coverage are more willing to try single-embryo transfer. Single-embryo transfer is much more common in Europe, where health insurance generally covers IVF procedures. Nevertheless, even in Europe only 20 percent to 25 percent of transfers are with a single embryo.

Fertility specialists may also feel pressure from couples to be aggressive. Some couples feel that after going through all of the preparation for an IVF cycle, they want the best chance to have a baby, and they accept the risk of having twins. Other couples are willing, if not eager, to have twins to complete their family more quickly or to ensure that their child has a sibling.

At Weill Cornell, single-embryo transfer is recommended for women who are below thirty-four years old, have a good egg yield at harvest, and have at least eight to ten healthy embryos on the third day after retrieval. This scenario is likely to yield healthy blastocysts with a high probability for implantation. Any woman who has already delivered a baby and/or has medical complications that may be exacerbated by a multiple pregnancy should undergo single-embryo transfer.

Genetic Testing of Embryos

With momentum building to transfer just one or two embryos, fertility clinics have begun to focus on choosing the one embryo that is most likely to succeed. Traditionally, embryos have been selected for transfer based on a visual examination of their morphology, that is, their shape, the number of cell divisions, and other physical factors. But many embryos that look great under the microscope have undetected chromosomal abnormalities, such as missing or extra chromosomes.

At Weill Cornell, the IVF team uses preimplantation genetic diagnosis (PGD) to select healthy embryos in couples who may have missing or extra chromosomes or who may be at risk of having a child with a genetic disease. For PGD, one or two cells are removed from the developing embryo for analysis. This allows the IVF team to identify embryos that do not carry the gene for certain inherited diseases such as cystic fibrosis and sickle cell anemia. This capability greatly reduces the risk that these diseases will be passed on to children—and without significantly lowering pregnancy rates. (See Chapter 12 for more on PGD.)

Another screening tool is called comparative genomic hybridization (CGH), which is a genetic test that analyzes the chromosomes in an egg or embryo before the transfer stage of an IVF cycle. Healthy humans carry forty-six chromosomes—twenty-three chromosomes contributed by the egg and twenty-three chromosomes contributed by the sperm. Eggs begin their development process with the full complement of forty-six chromosomes, but half of them are shed into a small genetic bundle known as the *polar body*.

CGH can screen the chromosomes from up to five cells taken from a blastocyst or analyze the genetic quality of eggs by examining DNA in the polar body. The test results take up to a week, so blastocysts are frozen and then thawed for implantation in a later IVF cycle. This allows the selection of a normal embryo, and some clinics have reported high pregnancy rates using this procedure. However, the polar body mirrors the chromosomes of the egg only, so CGH tests for chromosomal abnormalities derived from the egg, not the sperm.

Newer technology using gene chip analysis can now be used to screen embryos within two days. The jury is still out as to whether genetic testing increases pregnancy success rates. So far, genetic testing has not been used successfully to decrease the risk of multiple pregnancies.

Poor Responders

Sometimes a woman doesn't respond optimally to ovulation-inducing drugs. Blood tests and ultrasound exams may reveal insufficient follicle growth, or her eggs may be too immature to become fertilized. Women over age thirty-seven and those with a diminished ovarian reserve (a lower number of eggs) tend to have a poor response to hormone treatments. In these scenarios, increasing the dosage of ovarian stimulating drugs may have limited benefits. Nevertheless, novel treatment protocols have been developed for these women who are poor responders (see Chapter 12).

Poor responders under age thirty-five, especially when their baseline FSH levels are marginally elevated, present a particular challenge. Dr. Rosenwaks has devised a treatment for this group of women. He treats them with an estradiol patch and GnRH antagonist suppression in the luteal phase of the previous menstrual cycle, followed by a high dose of ovulation-inducing drugs. This protocol seems to lead to slightly higher implantation rates and pregnancy rates.

Women who don't respond to hormone treatments or those with breast cancer who should avoid estrogen therapy may consider an unstimulated, natural IVF cycle. The first successful IVF baby, England's Louise Brown, was born after retrieval of one egg from a natural menstrual cycle. A breast cancer survivor may also take the antiestrogen drug tamoxifen (Nolvadex) to recruit more than one follicle in what has proven to be a seemingly safe IVF procedure. Other unique protocols have been investigated for breast cancer patients who should not be exposed to high levels of estrogens. Letrozole (Femara) is a drug that inhibits estradiol production while allowing FSH to promote follicle and egg development. It has been used successfully in breast cancer patients.

The Age Effect

As we've mentioned, age is a critical factor in limiting a woman's chances of conceiving. That holds true for IVF success as well. Older women tend to have fewer eggs available for retrieval in an IVF cycle. And although a woman's age does not affect the egg's ability to become fertilized, it has a tremendous impact on the embryo's ability to implant in her uterus.

A woman's age is the single most important variable affecting success rates, particularly in IVF, with the number of pregnancies decreasing sharply after age forty. As women get older, we see increasing difficulties in obtaining positive responses to our treatments and techniques, in addition to a higher rate of miscarriages. In our practice, more than half of our patients who are women younger than age thirty-five take home babies. Between ages thirty-six and thirty-nine, about 40 percent of our women patients have babies. We don't shy away from difficult-to-treat couples—in one third of our couples, the woman is over age forty, and about one quarter of our female patients have a diminished ovarian reserve. For women age forty and up, more than 20 percent of our couples become pregnant.

IVF can overcome infertility in young women but not for those over forty. A large study by Boston researchers shows that IVF treatments often work for women under thirty-five but success rates are much lower for those over forty. The researchers followed more than six thousand women who went for their first fresh-embryo, nondonor IVF cycle from 2000 through 2005 at a single center and calculated their cumulative live-birth rates, that is, their chances of taking home a baby after multiple IVF cycles, not just one cycle. After six cycles of IVF, women younger than thirty-five had cumulative live-birth rates of between 65 percent and 86 percent, which is about the same as is observed in the general population. However, cumulative live-birth rates were only 23 percent to 42 percent of those aged forty and older. It should be emphasized that these results apply to a single clinic. Other institutions have reported higher pregnancy rates in older women.

Frozen Embryos

. . . .

In Cheri's second IVF attempt, the thirty-four-year-old had sixteen eggs retrieved and fertilized with sperm from her husband Tim, a forty-year-old golf pro. Four embryos were transferred, and the one that implanted successfully eventually became their daughter, Emily, who is now eight years old. "We were left with a dozen frozen embryos in storage, and we still can't decide what to do with them," says Tim. "Do we throw them out? Some people have funerals, but we're not there. Do we donate them? I have a moral issue with that because I would feel obligated if anything bad happened to the children created from the embryos."

Their solution: "We decided not to decide," says Tim. "We've had this discussion every six months for years. That gives us the most options."

. . . .

Most IVF clinics have embraced freezing embryos as a way to enhance a couple's chances of achieving a pregnancy. Better ovulation-induction protocols now allow Dr. Rosenwaks to harvest ten or more mature eggs from a woman in one cycle of hormonal stimulation. Before embryo freezing techniques became routinely available, a woman producing so many eggs would be forced to limit the number of eggs to be inseminated or to discard healthy embryos, since only a few were transferred to the uterus after being fertilized.

Freezing embryos allows couples to have several IVF treatment cycles from the same egg collection, reducing the number of times the ovaries are stimulated and therefore reducing the costs. The most costly part of an IVF cycle is the ovulation-induction, egg-retrieval, and fertilization stages. Frozen embryos can also be used during a natural-cycle IVF without any hormonal stimulation. Natural-cycle replacement is an easier procedure, and Dr. Rosenwaks recommends this for a woman who ovulates regularly and normally.

The thawed embryos are placed into the uterus three to five days after ovulation in exactly the same way as fresh embryos. The transfer is timed to the stage of development of the embryo. Embryos frozen at the eight-cell stage are transferred earlier than those frozen at the blastocyst stage. In a natural cycle, embryos frozen on the third day at the eight-cell stage will be thawed and transferred three days after the LH surge, while embryos frozen at the blastocyst stage will be transferred five days after ovulation. When a programmed cycle is used, day-3 embryos are transferred three days after initiating progesterone treatment.

About 75 percent of frozen embryos survive thawing at Weill Cornell. Our pregnancy rates are slightly higher—above 50 percent—when blastocysts are thawed and transferred compared to earlier-stage embryos.

Initially there were some concerns about the health of children born to women who had frozen embryos transferred, but now we know these children are just as normal as those conceived with fresh embryos. There's even some evidence that frozen embryos are healthier than fresh embryos. A Danish study found that women implanted with frozen embryos had babies who weighed slightly more than those implanted with fresh embryos, and they also had fewer multiple births. The reason for the differences is probably that only top-quality embryos survive the freezing and thawing process and are therefore healthier.

Embryos can remain viable for decades if they are frozen properly. Before freezing embryos, Dr. Rosenwaks asks the couple to sign a consent agreement stating that frozen embryos are the joint property of the couple. Before a woman reaches fifty-five, the frozen embryos must be thawed and implanted, donated to research, or disposed of. When the woman reaches fifty-five, the frozen embryos become the property of the Weill Cornell IVF team.

Couples also have the option to donate frozen embryos to another couple. In this case the Weill Cornell IVF program must comply with New York State tissue banking mandates and federal guidelines that require infectious disease testing within at least thirty days of egg retrieval. The donating couple must undergo genetic testing and a psychological evaluation.

In the Future

Several fertility teams are working on powerful new technologies that can screen chromosomes to look for inherited diseases with great accuracy and simplicity or can examine the chemical fingerprint of a woman's eggs to predict IVF success. Others are looking at ways to provide a clear view of the uterus during embryo transfer.

Genetic and Chemical Fingerprints

British researchers have devised a way to examine an embryo's DNA fingerprint and provide much fuller information about its genetic quality. The new technique, called *karyomapping*, analyzes chromosomes for almost any known genetic disease. The researchers take a single cell from an eight-cell embryo as well as DNA samples from the couple and the couple's parents and, if need be, also from a child affected by a genetic disorder. Then they compare all of the family members' DNA samples to look at 300,000 specific DNA markers. From this comparison, they create a map of the family's genetics. The researchers may also be able to use the test to improve the couple's chances of pregnancy by selecting embryos that stand the best chance of developing normally.

The British researchers are validating karyomapping by testing it alongside conventional PGD so they can check the results. It would make genetic screening much more straightforward but it could become controversial. Besides mutations that cause serious disorders such as cystic fibrosis, muscular dystrophy, and Huntington disease, the test could also reveal an embryo's future susceptibility to a host of other medical conditions, such as heart disease or cancer. That would raise questions of privacy, since it would reveal sensitive health information about the children born after karyomapping.

In another development, Stanford University researchers have come up with a way to profile a woman's embryos to determine which ones are more likely to result in pregnancies. This technique may provide an instantaneous snapshot of the physiology of an embryo using metabolomic profiling. Metabolomic profiling reveals trace molecules remaining after an array of cellular processes in the embryo. Previous studies have shown that this type of profiling can be used to identify unique biomarkers left behind by embryos in culture. It should be emphasized, however, that this technology is experimental and has yet to be proven clinically useful.

Early investigations have established a correlation between the number of particular trace elements left behind by an early embryo, an embryo's viability, and how likely a woman is to become pregnant. If future studies confirm these results, the test could someday be used to predict the success of IVF and help determine which eggs should be selected for fertilization or to be frozen.

Imaging during Embryo Transfer

With all of the significant advancements in IVF, the one step that has seen little change is the embryo transfer procedure. Typically, an embryo transfer is performed using a "blind" technique, as the fertility specialist inserts a thin catheter through the vagina and into the uterus. Several groups have proposed using fiber-optic technology to allow direct visualization of a woman's anatomy during an embryo transfer. These techniques are experimental and their superiority has not yet been demonstrated.

Some fertility specialists use two-dimensional and three-dimensional ultrasound to guide embryo transfers. Dr. Rosenwaks uses ultrasound guidance of the embryo transfer only for difficult placements. A previously performed mock transfer informs him whether he may encounter difficulty during the embryo transfer.

· · · · · · ·

One of the most sophisticated IVF techniques is the manipulation of sperm and eggs using very fine microtools. Using these tiny tools, a highly trained specialist can puncture the outer layers of an egg and inject a single sperm inside in what's known as an ICSI procedure. The next chapter shows how this technique has revolutionized the treatment of male infertility.

Take-Home Messages

- You may be a candidate for IVF if you have tubal factor infertility, the man has very poor sperm quality or no sperm in his ejaculate, the woman is age thirty-seven or older with diminished ovarian reserve or has untreatable endometriosis, you have a diagnosis of unexplained infertility or antisperm antibodies, or you carry genetic abnormalities.
- Several hormone preparations are available to develop more than one follicle in an IVF cycle.
- The embryo transfer is a simple, short outpatient procedure with no anesthesia.
- An individualized ovarian stimulation protocol can reduce the incidence of overstimulation of the ovaries.
- In young women, only one or two healthy embryos are transferred.
- The woman's age is the single most important factor affecting IVF success.
- Frozen embryos allow you to have several IVF treatment cycles after a single egg collection.

Eleven

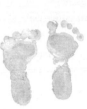

Am I a Candidate for ICSI?
When to Do Intracytoplasmic Sperm Injection

· · · · · · · · · ·

Ten years after his divorce, Hank, then a forty-four-year-old computer consultant, met and married Nicole, a thirty-four-year-old banker. They wanted children together, so Hank contacted Dr. Goldstein to reverse the vasectomy his first wife had requested. During the reversal operation, Dr. Goldstein aspirated sperm from Hank's epididymis and froze them in case he needed them later.

The vasectomy reversal was successful, but Hank's sperm had poor motility, so Dr. Goldstein suggested they try an in vitro fertilization (IVF) procedure with injection of one of Hank's sperm directly into one of Nicole's eggs. Nicole took fertility drugs to induce multiple eggs. After harvesting her eggs, "they thawed my sperm sample, pulled out some winners, placed them in a solution to slow them down, and selected the strongest ones. Then they put the eggs together with the sperm," says Hank.

Nicole had the procedure, and one of the three embryos that were transferred survived. "We have a photo of the transferred embryos in Judy's baby book. One of them is her," says Hank. "Judy is a marvelous eight-year-old child. It does make you stop and be grateful. When something is so hard to get, you appreciate it a little more."

· · · · · · · · · ·

Assisted reproductive technologies (ART) have advanced to the point where a single sperm can be physically injected into an egg. This procedure, called intracytoplasmic sperm injection (ICSI), has dramatically changed the options available for even the most severe male-factor infertility. Because of this technique, 90 percent of all infertile men have the potential to conceive their own genetic child.

ICSI has become the single most important development in ART since the arrival of IVF. In particular, ICSI has revolutionized the treatment of infertility for couples who do not succeed with IVF. In our hands, ICSI procedures for severe male-factor infertility result in pregnancy rates of more than 50 percent in young women. In fact, the success rates of ICSI cycles are more dependent on the age of the female partner than the severity of the male factor. As we continue to make advancements with this technique, it becomes possible for any man who has even a single sperm in his ejaculate or a few sperm in his testicles to achieve fertilization and produce healthy offspring. ICSI continues to redefine the limits of male sterility.

The first babies were born through ICSI in 1992. Since then, hundreds of thousands of ICSI births have occurred. Using ICSI, even couples with severe infertility can now achieve a pregnancy and have a baby. In fact, the pregnancy and birth rates for problematic cases treated with ICSI just about equal those of couples with normal sperm and eggs who use conventional IVF. And there are now almost as many cycles of ICSI each year as there are conventional IVF cycles.

When to Do ICSI

Selecting a single sperm to be injected directly into a woman's egg is an effective option for a man with a very low sperm count or if his sperm cannot reach the egg successfully. Most often ICSI is indicated when a man has poor sperm quality. This means he has less than half a million moving sperm in his ejaculate; less than 1 percent of normally shaped sperm; poor sperm motility; a zero sperm count (azoospermia), but sperm can be surgically retrieved from his epididymis or testicles; round-headed sperm that lack an enzyme cap; or sperm that fail to fertilize his partner's eggs.

ICSI bypasses many of the barriers that can interfere with male fertility. These include antisperm antibodies stuck to sperm, abnormal ejaculation, azoospermia due to obstruction of the sperm-carrying ducts, a decreased quantity and quality of sperm, and even nonobstructive azoospermia (NOA), where there are no sperm in the semen but a few sperm can be extracted microsurgically directly from the testicles (a procedure called testicular sperm extraction, or TESE). The only requirement is one good sperm.

We also apply ICSI when a woman has certain persistent fertility problems. ICSI may be indicated for women who have too few eggs harvested, for women where the protective coating of the eggs (the zona pellucida) is too thick, or for any situation where the eggs cannot be penetrated naturally, for example, due to high levels of antisperm antibodies.

Couples with one partner infected with the hepatitis C virus or human immunodeficiency virus are also good candidates for ICSI. ICSI virtually avoids the interaction of eggs with the seminal fluid that sperm is normally mixed with at the time of ejaculation and reduces the risk of viral exposure. Some couples in this situation choose intrauterine insemination (IUI), but ICSI has a higher success rate than IUI, takes fewer attempts to achieve a pregnancy, and reduces the unaffected partner's exposure to the virus. And the treatment is relatively safe. There have been no reports of unaffected partners becoming infected with these viruses after IVF or ICSI procedures.

The ICSI Procedure

The ICSI procedure usually begins like a conventional IVF cycle. The woman takes daily ovulation-inducing drugs for about one to two weeks with the aim of producing more than one egg. Ultrasound scans track her follicle development, and when the follicles are ripe, she comes in to the fertility clinic for retrieval of the eggs. Under sedation, the eggs are retrieved with ultrasound guidance through her vagina. Then, instead of mixing many sperm with the eggs in the laboratory, as with IVF, a highly trained specialist delicately carries out the ICSI procedure.

Usually, the male partner collects the sperm on the morning when his female partner undergoes the egg retrieval. The sperm are washed and undergo a motility-enhancing process in the laboratory. Then they are deposited in a viscous solution to slow their motion. This allows the specialist to visualize, select, and aspirate a single sperm into a microneedle. The sperm is then immobilized by crushing the tail, which enhances the chance of fertilization. Using a high-powered microscope, the specialist holds the egg on the end of a very tiny glass tube and injects the single sperm directly into the center of the egg.

Intracytoplasmic Sperm Injection (ICSI)

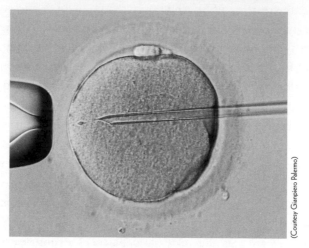

(Courtesy Gianpiero Palermo)

Once each of the eggs is injected with one sperm apiece, the eggs are incubated for sixteen to eighteen hours in a special culture medium. Then the eggs are examined for possible damage during their handling with the microtools. Using a meticulous technique under the most optimal conditions, about 95 percent of the injected eggs survive the procedure at Weill Cornell. The fertilized eggs are cultured for three to five days, and the embryos or blastocysts are transferred back to the woman's uterus with a catheter placed through her cervix.

With expanded indications for ICSI, it has become the standard insemination method to fertilize an egg in most large fertility clinics. We now perform ICSI in 70 percent of all ART cycles at Weill Cornell.

How ICSI Compares to IVF

Unlike conventional IVF, which incubates about one hundred thousand moving sperm with an egg, ICSI requires only one sperm per egg. ICSI procedures achieve high fertilization and pregnancy rates that compare favorably to those of conventional IVF among couples without male-factor infertility. There was a suggestion in early studies that embryos from ICSI were compromised. However, more recent, larger studies show that the embryos that form from ICSI are just as healthy as those that arise from IVF.

There is little difference in the implantation rates, pregnancy rates, and delivery rates between the two procedures.

Over the last fifteen years at Weill Cornell, we have performed more than twenty-five thousand ART cycles. Just more than one third of those ART cycles have been conventional IVF, and the rest have been ICSI. The average age of couples is the same for both IVF and ICSI—thirty-seven for our female patients and forty for our male patients.

Both ICSI and IVF yield very similar results. For the nearly ten thousand couples we have treated with ICSI, fertilization rates with a variety of types of sperm collection are approximately 75 percent to 80 percent. Success rates are dependent on the female partner's age. Women younger than thirty-four can expect pregnancy rates of about 50 percent per cycle.

The risks to the woman of IVF with ICSI are no different from regular IVF. Commonly reported side effects of stimulating the ovaries include tiredness, breast tenderness, pelvic discomfort, and mood swings. The most serious complication is ovarian hyperstimulation syndrome (OHSS) caused by the ovulation-inducing drugs. This syndrome can lead to the development of severe ovarian enlargement, fluid accumulation, abdominal swelling, and respiratory and kidney problems. In rare cases it can be fatal.

The ICSI procedure itself—injecting a sperm into an egg—may compromise the protective outer layer surrounding the egg. The sperm preparation and manipulation may cause immediate disintegration of the egg or may lead to abnormal fertilization. Abnormally fertilized eggs are not transferred. Because of all of these possibilities, in the past we strongly recommended that when a woman became pregnant after ICSI, she underwent amniocentesis or chorionic villus sampling as well as thorough ultrasound exams of the fetus throughout her pregnancy. More recently we have suggested she follow similar guidelines recommended after standard IVF.

The risks of embryo transfer are the same as those with IVF. Bacterial or viral infections may occur, since the catheter used to transfer the embryo has to pass through the cervix and is a potential source of infection.

Once fertilization is achieved with ICSI, pregnancy success rates depend upon the female partner's age and are similar to the success rates observed with standard IVF. IVF with ICSI has become the treatment of choice for many older women, particularly those who have only a few good eggs available upon retrieval. Importantly, ICSI requires that the egg be cleared (freed) from its surrounding granulosa (nourishing) cells, allowing the embryologist to better evaluate its quality and maturity. In conventional IVF, about 30 percent of eggs fail to become fertilized due to either sperm defects or eggs that have not matured enough or are abnormal. ICSI has been proven to be an effective method to improve pregnancy rates among couples who have previously had unsuccessful IVF cycles because of poor fertilization.

ICSI Offspring

Some early studies questioned whether children born after ICSI developed normally. But follow-up studies at Weill Cornell of five-year-old ICSI children show no problems in terms of psychological or physical development. The early development of the children born using ICSI is the same as with IVF.

Of the nearly seven thousand babies born after ICSI at Weill Cornell, only 3 percent have had birth defects, the same incidence observed in our IVF babies. This percentage is no greater than that of the general population.

ICSI itself does not induce chromosomal abnormalities, but the children born through ICSI may be at risk of inheriting genetic defects found in sperm. Infertile men tend to have a higher incidence of chromosomal abnormalities as well as too many or too few chromosomes in their sperm. From 5 percent to 15 percent of men with severely low sperm counts have a Y chromosome microdeletion. This mutation is passed along to their male children but not their female children, because only the boys inherit the father's Y chromosome. Another 10 percent to 15 percent of men with severe male-factor infertility have chromosomal abnormalities.

Men who are born without any vas deferens, a condition known as congenital bilateral absence of the vas deferens (CBAVD), may have sperm aspirated from the tubules of their epididymis or from their testicles for ICSI. These men often have mutations in a gene associated with cystic fibrosis. There are some studies that suggest that boys conceived through IVF with ICSI have a higher incidence of congenital abnormalities of the genitourinary system, primarily hypospadias, where the opening of the urethra comes out of the shaft, not the end of the penis, and undescended testicles. These conditions are both correctable.

Sperm Aspiration

ICSI was originally designed to treat extremely poor sperm quality or cases in which eggs failed to fertilize with IVF. ICSI has also become an important, if not the only, option for the one hundred thousand couples in whom a man's sperm is perfectly healthy but can't get out of the epididymis or where the man has CBAVD. At Weill Cornell, we have pioneered techniques in sperm aspiration that extract sperm either from the ducts leading from the testicle (vas deferens or epididymis) or from the testicle itself. These sperm can then be used in ICSI procedures.

Men who have an obstruction in the vas deferens or epididymis due to a previous infection, scrotal surgery, or failed vasectomy reversal can also benefit from ICSI. We can either aspirate and then freeze sperm from these tubes at the time of the microsurgical procedure to reverse the obstruction or perform the aspiration (and use the fresh sperm) at the time the female partner undergoes an IVF retrieval. With the advent of ICSI, it became possible to obtain a high fertilization rate by injecting these fully motile sperm directly into eggs.

The most effective sperm retrieval technique is called microsurgical epididymal sperm aspiration (MESA). The man is put under general anesthesia. A small cut is made into the scrotum, the ducts of the epididymis are exposed under a microscope, a tiny microknife is used to open the epididymis, and the sperm are aspirated into a tiny glass tube. The sperm are placed in a special culture medium and frozen. The urologist can extract enough sperm in a single operation for at least four or five attempts at IVF or ICSI. This operation is less extensive than a vasectomy reversal operation, but it does require anesthesia and an incision in the scrotum. The sperm aspiration procedure takes about one to two hours. Our pregnancy rate using MESA is about 63 percent.

The specific complications of MESA include wound infection, hematoma, and pain. These occur in less than one in a thousand cases.

Dr. Goldstein can also obtain sperm directly from the testicles in what is known as testicular for sperm aspiration (TESA). The man undergoes either a local anesthesia or light general anesthesia, then Dr. Goldstein puts a needle directly into the testicle to aspirate the sperm. Because far fewer sperm can be obtained this way and because they don't always survive freezing and thawing, this procedure should be done simultaneously with an IVF or ICSI attempt, and the sperm aspiration is coordinated with the woman's egg retrieval. Testicular sperm have not had a chance to mature, so pregnancy rates are lower with testicular sperm (about 25 percent) than with sperm aspirated from the epididymis or the vas deferens.

Testicular Epididymal Sperm Aspiration (TESA)

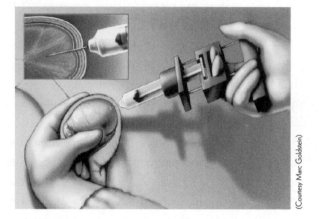

(Courtesy Marc Goldstein)

The specific complications of TESA are similar to MESA and also include injury to the testicle's blood vessels from the blind needle aspiration. In rare instances, this causes the testicle to atrophy (diminish in size).

We have performed more than two thousand ICSI procedures at Weill Cornell using surgically retrieved sperm. Our fertilization rates are still high (60 percent), though not quite as high as that with ejaculated sperm (75 percent). There's no real difference in fertilization rates when sperm are aspirated from an obstructed epididymis and injected immediately and when they have been frozen and thawed later on, as long as the sperm survive the freeze and thaw.

For men who have a vasectomy reversal on at least one side, we usually do not recommend sperm aspiration at the time of surgery because our success rate for return of sperm to the semen is 99.5 percent. Because vasectomy reversal yields pregnancy rates between 50 percent and 70 percent through natural conception, we usually recommend sperm aspiration as a secondary procedure. On the other hand, if the woman has a fertility factor that requires an ART procedure, then we recommend ICSI with aspirated sperm instead of a vasectomy reversal.

However, if Dr. Goldstein needs to do a reversal that connects the epididymis to the vas deferens on both sides, the success rate for return of sperm drops to 80 percent. If a man needs this more extensive procedure, we recommend sperm aspiration at the time of surgery. These sperm are frozen and become available for future IVF or ICSI cycles in the event that the surgery to repair the blockage is not successful. If live sperm are present but the woman is not getting pregnant, then we can use ICSI with ejaculated sperm even if the sperm are low in number.

Testicular Extraction

Sperm can also be extracted from the testicles of men who have azoospermia and no blockages. The preferred procedure for these men with NOA is called microdissection TESE, a procedure that was developed by Weill Cornell researchers. TESE is best performed fresh at the time of the woman's egg retrieval. Usually the man undergoes regional or general anesthesia, then the urologist makes a long incision in the scrotum to access the four hundred U-shaped seminiferous tubules in each testicle. Using a high-powered operating microscope, he searches for the larger tubules that are more likely to contain sperm. A tiny section of each of these tubules is microsurgically removed, and the sperm are located. The sperm are examined by the embryologist, and if they are alive, are immediately injected into the female's eggs using ICSI. Any extra sperm are frozen and preserved for future use.

This type of microsurgical sperm retrieval is the procedure of choice for men with inflammation of the scrotum, men who have had previous surgery on the scrotum, or those who have small testicles. The likelihood of finding sperm during TESE depends upon the type of NOA the man has. Sperm can be retrieved successfully about 60 percent to 70 percent of the time from men with poor sperm formation, about 50 percent of the time from men who have arrested sperm maturation, and about 25 percent of the time from those with Sertoli-cell-only pattern on previous biopsy.

Using TESE combined with ICSI, we achieved the first live births in couples where the male partner had Klinefelter syndrome. This syndrome, which affects about one in five hundred or six hundred men, occurs when the man is born with an extra X chromosome. For reasons that are still unclear, this can dramatically lower the number of sperm in the testicles. The sperm counts for these men are so low that they were long considered sterile and untreatable. However, they may have patches of sperm in their testicles that can be extracted with TESE. This has given new hope to men who otherwise would never have been able to become biological fathers.

The specific complications of TESE are the same as for MESA. The microsurgical technique avoids injuring the blood vessels on the surface of the testicles, which can occur if the surgeon extracts sperm without micro-surgery. Because the numbers of sperm retrieved from the testicles of men with NOA are so low compared with men who have obstruction, TESE is best performed at the time of or one day before egg retrieval, so that fresh sperm can be used. If sperm are frozen, many don't survive the thaw.

In Vitro Maturation

A procedure called in vitro maturation (IVM) may allow women to un-dergo IVF without the discomfort, risk, and expense of daily hormone injections, although it's somewhat less effective than IVF. In IVM, immature eggs are harvested from the ovaries without the use of ovulation-inducing drugs and matured in the laboratory before being fertilized with ICSI.

The IVM technique is challenging because the follicles that contain the immature eggs are less than half the size of follicles containing mature eggs. This makes them harder to spot and harder to retrieve. They have to be removed with a collection needle placed at the correct angle and nurtured in special nutrient and hormone solution before they are fertilized and transferred into the uterus.

IVM Procedure

The IVM procedure begins with a woman having a vaginally inserted ul-trasound scan between days 2 and 4 of her menstrual cycle to count the number of follicles in her ovaries. The ultrasound is repeated between days 6 and 10 to check for natural ovulation. If she has one dominant follicle, then fewer immature eggs can be harvested, and either the cycle is canceled or she becomes a candidate for natural-cycle IVF combined with IVM.

The woman receives an injection of human chorionic gonadotropin (hCG) thirty-six hours before the immature eggs are retrieved, which is usually between days 8 and 11 of her cycle. Most often, the woman is placed under sedation to reduce her movement during the egg retrieval. The immature eggs are placed in tubes containing specialized media to help the eggs mature. Once the eggs become mature, each one is injected with a single sperm and cultured for several additional days. The embryos that develop are transferred on day 2 or 3 after ICSI.

If the endometrial lining is too thin on day 6 of the cycle, the woman takes estrogen to promote growth of the endometrium. On the day of the egg retrieval she starts taking estradiol, on the day of ICSI she starts taking progesterone, and she continues these drugs through the first three months to support her pregnancy.

IVM Candidates

The best candidates for IVM appear to be young women with large numbers of follicles, women with polycystic ovary syndrome (PCOS) who have not conceived after a handful of IVF cycles, and women who produce poor-quality embryos during conventional IVF. IVM may also be a possibility for egg donors as well as young women undergoing chemotherapy or radio-therapy for cancer treatments who need to reduce the lengthy fertility treat-ment time and the risks of hormonal stimulation and elevated estrogens, especially if they have estrogen-sensitive cancer (for example, breast cancer).

IVM has several advantages over IVF. IVM saves couples about $5,000 by eliminating the need for expensive fertility drugs, and with fewer hormone injections, there's less need for monitoring and fewer side effects.

The trade-off is that the success rate for IVM is at least 20 percent lower than conventional IVF or ICSI. Older women and those with high blood levels of follicle-stimulating hormone (FSH), which is an indication of a low number of follicles, are least likely to become pregnant after IVM.

In the Future

Choosing one healthy sperm becomes crucial to ICSI success. In a natural conception, only the fittest and healthiest sperm makes the arduous journey to the egg. ICSI bypasses this natural selection barrier, so the chances of a genetically abnormal sperm fertilizing an egg are higher. A new test for sperm DNA damage could help select the best sperm for a single-sperm injection.

Sperm Quality Test

Researchers have developed a new way to examine the quality of a sperm without damaging it, making it possible to determine whether the sperm is healthy enough to fertilize an egg. An individual sperm's DNA properties are identified by the pattern of the vibrations it emits after it is captured in two highly focused beams of laser light. The technology, called *Raman spectroscopy*, is used to label each sperm with a DNA-based quality score.

Recently, a new imaging technique that enhances the ability to evaluate sperm, called intracytoplasmic morphologically selected sperm injection (IMSI), has been reported to increase the ability to select the "best" sperm. IMSI may help increase pregnancy rates and reduce miscarriage rates compared to routine ICSI, but these findings need to be confirmed.

Although the sperm chosen for ICSI may appear quite normal, many of them may in fact have DNA damage, which can decrease the chances of pregnancy. An embryologist normally selects the best-looking sperm for injection by analyzing the sperm's shape under a microscope. A good sperm will appear to have a regular, oval head and a long, straight tail.

However, appearances can be deceiving. Many normal-looking sperm have DNA fragmentation. Many factors may contribute to sperm DNA fragmentation, including reproductive tract infection, age, smoking, exposure to air pollution, and abnormally high testicular temperature. It has been suggested that if damaged sperm are used, the chances of the woman miscarrying may be higher. The significance of DNA damage on pregnancies following ICSI is unclear. However, with conventional IVF or natural pregnancy, DNA fragmentation may be associated with increased miscarriages.

Numerous tests have been developed to screen sperm for DNA damage, but these tests destroy the sperm. This new test does not cause any damage to sperm, so if the sperm has good quality DNA, it can still be used in an IVF or ICSI procedure.

The new sperm-quality test could complement conventional semen analysis and help predict the risk of a miscarriage or enhance the chance of pregnancy success. Currently, the research is in a preclinical phase, and the test won't become available to couples for five years or more.

Take-Home Messages

- You may be a good candidate for ICSI if you have very poor-quality sperm.
- If you are a woman age thirty-seven or older, ICSI may be the preferred treatment if you have only a few mature eggs retrieved during IVF cycles.
- Children born using ICSI show no additional problems in terms of psychological or physical development, although some studies contradict these findings.
- Sperm can be extracted from the ducts leading from the testicle (vas deferens or epididymis) or from the testicle itself and then used in ICSI procedures.
- You may be a very good candidate for IVM if you are a young woman with a large number of follicles, have PCOS, and have not conceived after several IVF cycles.

Twelve

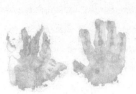

What Are My Other Options?
Strategies to Overcome Common Hurdles in IVF

· · · · · · · · · ·

"A urologist at another medical center told us we had enough sperm for intrauterine insemination," says Ben, a forty-six-year-old pilot. "But after six failed IUIs and one miscarriage, he suggested we move on to in vitro fertilization (IVF) at Weill Cornell. He was worried because my wife, Sarah, had just turned forty."

Dr. Goldstein examined Ben and felt a varicocele in his left testicle and another in his right one. That accounted for his poor semen quality. *"You don't want C-plus sperm if you can have A-grade sperm. Every factor is important,"* says Ben. Dr. Goldstein surgically removed the varicoceles as well as hydroceles on both sides.

In the meantime, Sarah started to prepare for an IVF cycle with intracytoplasmic sperm injection (ICSI) by taking fertility drugs to produce more than one egg. *"Every part of the IVF process is a guessing game. How many eggs are going to be retrieved? Will they be mature enough? How many will be fertilized successfully? How many implanted?"* says Ben, whose sperm were of good-enough quality one month after his operation to use in the ICSI procedure. Six of Sarah's eggs were retrieved, four were fertilized, and three were transferred. Then they received the crushing news that none had survived.

Three months later, they began a second cycle of IVF with ICSI with the addition of embryo co-culture. One month before the scheduled cycle, *"Dr. Rosenwaks scraped the lining of Sarah's uterus to gather some cells. When we did the IVF cycle the next month, he put those cells in with our three embryos to help*

them grow better. My sperm count had tripled and their motility and morphol-
ogy also increased," says Ben. "The two-week wait after the three embryos were
transferred was torture. Sarah was worried that it wouldn't work again after all of
the injections she had had to endure. I tried to encourage her, reminding her that
we had better sperm this time." Ben and Sarah have just found out that Sarah is
pregnant with their first child.

· · · · · · · · ·

The predominant reason why women age thirty-seven and older are less likely to conceive than younger women and have poor success with in vitro fertilization (IVF) relates to the genetic makeup of their eggs. Chromosomal abnormalities in older women are for the most part responsible for the lower implantation rates and higher miscarriage rates. As important a factor is that standard ovarian stimulation protocols yield fewer eggs and lower estradiol levels in women of advanced reproductive age. Consequently, several strategies have been devised in an effort to improve responses and the number of eggs retrieved.

When ovarian stimulation protocols fail to overcome age-related failures, egg donation is often the final option for many women who cannot use their own eggs. We discuss egg donation in full in Chapter 13.

Improved Ovarian Stimulation

· · · · · · · · ·

"I started to think about having kids at thirty-seven, and it took longer than I
expected," says Deborah. Her husband, Peter, age forty, had a low sperm count
due to two large varicoceles, which were surgically removed by Dr. Goldstein. "We
knew it would take a while for Peter's fertility to come back, so I sought out a fer-
tility doctor, who suggested we try IVF. I had a high initial FSH level and did not
respond well to the ovarian stimulation hormones. I had only one or two eggs, and
the IVF cycle was canceled," she says. The fertility doctor changed the stimulation
protocol, using megadoses in the next cycle, but Deborah still produced only two
eggs, and the IVF cycle was again canceled. "The doctor told me, 'At your age, you
should start thinking about an egg donor program,'" she recalls.

At that point, they went to see Dr. Rosenwaks. He discovered that Deborah
had uterine adhesions. She had surgery to remove the adhesions and then began
an IVF cycle under Dr. Rosenwaks's direction. "He prescribed a different protocol

because of my high FSH level. I wore an estradiol patch for five days before day 1 of the cycle. That brought down my FSH level on day 2," she says. Five of Deborah's eggs were retrieved, three were fertilized, and two embryos were transplanted, but she did not become pregnant. "We were disappointed, but I had produced more eggs, and a few of them had matured," she said. They tried another IVF cycle with Dr. Rosenwaks. "This time, I had three healthy embryos transplanted and I became pregnant!" says Deborah. "The difference in the stimulation protocol was significant." Their son, Earl, is now two years old.

Dr. Rosenwaks has been involved in developing ovarian stimulation protocols since the early days of IVF. He has been in the forefront in forging individualized ovarian stimulation strategies to optimize IVF success while reducing side effects and complications. In most instances, women who exhibit low ovarian responses to stimulation have low ovarian reserves. Typically, women who do not respond well to stimulation protocols have lower peak estradiol levels, fewer eggs retrieved, and fewer embryos available for transfer. This all combines to reduce their chances of becoming pregnant.

To overcome some of the problems in women age thirty-seven and older, several approaches can be undertaken, all aimed at optimizing response and IVF success rates. Suppression of gonadotropins by gonadotropin-releasing hormone (GnRH) agonists has been a convenient method for programming IVF cycles, but women of thirty-seven and older often have a lower ovarian response in suppressed cycles. Consequently, omitting GnRH agonists or lowering the dosage of GnRH agonists may improve the stimulation response. It is also as important to increase the dose of gonadotropins, primarily follicle-stimulating hormone (FSH), in the early part of stimulation to help to develop more follicles and improve IVF outcome. Other approaches include using a GnRH agonist "flare" protocol (see below) or using frequent microdoses of GnRH to increase the woman's FSH secretion, all aimed at promoting follicle development. Indeed, some women respond better to their own FSH than to recombinant or urinary FSH preparations. Simultaneous exposure to high levels of administered FSH after suppression of a woman's own FSH often results in recruitment of a higher number of mature follicles. Another method to increase a woman's own FSH is to treat her with clomiphene pills, later to be accompanied by gonadotropins.

Some women benefit from late-luteal-phase administration of estradiol or estradiol in combination with GnRH antagonists. This is done to decrease the previously observed rise in FSH, which could result in the early development of a single follicle. This approach is especially helpful in women who have marginally elevated day-3 FSH.

Stimulation Protocols Designed for the Poor Responder

Over the last decade, several protocols have been developed for women with diminished ovarian reserve who exhibit poor response to standard gonadotropin stimulation. These protocols endeavor to minimize ovarian suppression and maximize responsiveness. One approach involves omitting GnRH agonist suppression or reducing the GnRH agonist dose while maintaining a high gonadotropin (FSH) starting dose.

Another approach utilizes the GnRH agonist "flare" protocol in the beginning of the menstrual cycle. For this protocol, GnRH agonists are administered twice daily, beginning on day 2 of the cycle—taking advantage of the initial GnRH agonist stimulatory effect on FSH secretion. The increased natural FSH is then complemented with high doses of FSH beginning two to three days later (on day 4 or 5 of the cycle), while continuing the twice-daily GnRH agonist. The agonist dosage can be reduced in a "microflare" approach.

In patients who exhibit marginally elevated FSH levels, we can pretreat with estradiol patches or oral contraceptive pills to suppress the precycle FSH rise. In poor responders, it is advantageous to avoid any pretreatment with GnRH agonist or oral contraceptives. These women benefit from starting FSH at high doses in the second day of the cycle and using GnRH antagonists to suppress any LH surges on the fourth or fifth day of stimulation. This approach avoids early suppression of the pituitary. The advantages of GnRH antagonist protocols are fewer injections and a shorter duration of stimulation compared to "microflare" regimens.

The side effects of these drugs are the same as those outlined in Chapter 10.

Ovarian Reserve Blood Test

A blood test can also provide information about the number of eggs in the ovaries. A hormone called anti-Müllerian hormone (AMH) is produced by follicles in the ovary. A higher AMH level indicates a higher number of follicles and eggs in the ovaries. As a woman gets older and the number of eggs in her ovaries decreases, the AMH levels also start to decrease.

AMH levels can be used to predict a woman's response to ovarian stimulation. In fact, we can determine which woman will have a higher or lower response by measuring her AMH levels at any time during her menstrual cycle. This allows Dr. Rosenwaks to choose a high or low FSH dosage even before the woman begins her treatment. FSH levels along with AMH concentrations can help a couple decide on whether to proceed with IVF, particularly if their previous IVF cycles have failed. Nevertheless, no hormonal marker of ovarian reserve is an absolute determinant of success or failure with IVF.

Currently, the test for AMH levels can be used to tailor the dose of fertility drugs in IVF to avoid overstimulation of the ovaries. But in the future its main use may be to help a woman with a reduced egg count make earlier fertility choices.

Endometrial-Cell Co-culture

IVF with endometrial-cell co-culture is a special technique for couples with poor embryo quality. This technique creates a more natural environment for the embryo to develop in. Endometrial-cell co-culture takes advantage of the woman's own cells to help embryos grow stronger. Embryos are grown in a culture medium along with cells from the lining of her uterus (the endometrium) to condition the embryo for transplantation. Weill Cornell researchers refined this technique using the woman's own endometrial cells rather than cells from animals. The result is improved IVF success rates for women whose previous IVF or ICSI attempts have failed. Repeated attempts at IVF with endometrial-cell co-culture have yielded higher success rates in women who have failed IVF due to poor embryo quality.

During a woman's menstrual cycle before a planned IVF cycle, an endometrial biopsy is performed during the mid-to-late luteal phase of the cycle. Cells from the endometrium are separated out, cultured in a special medium, and then frozen for later use.

When the couple begins an IVF cycle, the endometrial cells are thawed and the day-old embryos are placed on top of the mother's cells. The embryo and endometrial cells are co-cultured for two days, and then the embryo is transplanted using the standard method for IVF.

No one knows exactly how co-culturing works, but the endometrial cells seem to improve embryo development by releasing growth factors or possibly by absorbing toxins. We have noted that co-cultured embryos have slightly enhanced growth and appear healthier.

Our studies at Weill Cornell show that embryo co-culture helps women who have poor embryo quality or whose embryos fail to implant. This co-culture technique increases the number of blastomeres (the cells within the embryos) and decreases the amount of embryo fragmentation. As much as three quarters of embryos created through IVF contain cellular fragments. A high fragmentation rate diminishes an embryo's ability to implant.

Embryo co-culture enhances implantation and pregnancy rates. Our pregnancy rates with embryo co-culture approach those of conventional IVF in these challenging couples, even in couples who have seen several cycles fail.

There are no increased risks of birth defects with embryo co-culture. The risks appear to be similar to those observed with conventional IVF or ICSI cycles.

Assisted Hatching

There is another IVF technique designed to enhance implantation of embryos. Known as assisted hatching, this microsurgical procedure is performed in the embryology laboratory on embryos before they are transferred during an IVF cycle.

About one week after fertilization, an embryo naturally "hatches," that is, sheds its shell like outer layer (zona pellucida), to allow it to attach to the uterus. If the embryo is unable to hatch, it fails to implant. If need be, we can assist the hatching process to facilitate implantation and rescue embryos with abnormalities in their outer layers.

At Weill Cornell, an embryologist uses an acid solution to make a small opening in the embryo's outer layer. Other fertility clinics may use a laser to make the opening. The embryologist holds the embryo on the end of a very thin glass tube and gently applies the solution to a small area of the embryo's outer layer to create a tiny hole. After assisted hatching, the embryo is transferred according to its developmental stage.

Women may be good candidates for assisted hatching if they produce embryos with a thick or oddly shaped outer shell, have embryos with a high percentage of fragmentation within the embryo cells, or have not become pregnant within several IVF cycles. Embryos that exhibit normal morphology and little fragmentation do not benefit from assisted hatching.

Assisted hatching has been used on thousands of embryos, and although none of them have been destroyed, there is potential for harm occurring during the manipulation leading to damage of individual cells. Single cells of the embryo are damaged in less than 1 percent of cases, and when this occurs, it does not appear to affect the development of the growing embryo.

Although unlikely, assisted hatching may present unknown risks to the embryo. The breach created in the protective layer in the embryo may predispose the embryo to bacterial or other infections since the catheter used for embryo transfer goes through the cervix and may be a potential source of infection.

It should be emphasized that assisted hatching should be used selectively on embryos with poor morphology.

Preimplantation Genetic Diagnosis

PGD testing can be performed either at the time of insemination or ICSI or after an egg has been fertilized in vitro but before the resulting embryo is transferred to the uterus. The test results provide information about the genetic status of embryos to help ensure that only embryos free of problems are transferred. PGD can detect whether the embryo has too many or too few chromosomes or has a single-gene defect such as cystic fibrosis, Tay-Sachs disease, or sickle cell disease. Couples who are carriers of severe genetic disorders can minimize the risk of their baby being born with the disorder or having to make the difficult decision to abort the pregnancy.

Our research shows that as women age, they tend to have more chromosome abnormalities in their embryos. This increase or decrease in chromosomes is independent of the way an older woman's embryos look. A large proportion of normal-looking embryos actually have missing or extra chromosomes. About two thirds of the women who undergo PGD testing at Weill Cornell are older or have had repeated miscarriages or IVF failures. Using PGD, we can analyze the number of chromosomes in their embryos, then select and transfer normal embryos to help these couples achieve high implantation rates and lower miscarriage rates. This type of PGD is popularly called preimplantation genetic screening (PGS).

On day 3 of a woman's cycle, we remove one cell from the developing embryo using microsurgery. The one cell gently sucked out of the embryo is analyzed for genetic flaws. The embryo is placed back in culture and incubated for the one or two days it takes to get the results of the genetic test. A healthy embryo will continue to develop, and on day 5 we transfer the embryo (now a blastocyst) as in a routine IVF procedure. If there's a technical delay in the PGD test results beyond day 6, a healthy blastocyst may be frozen for transfer in a future IVF cycle.

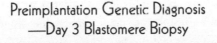

Preimplantation Genetic Diagnosis —Day 3 Blastomere Biopsy

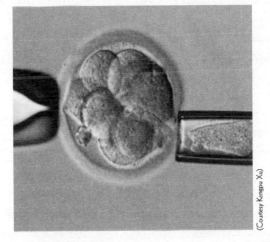

(Courtesy Kengpu Xu)

Babies born after PGD have the same birth weight as babies born through conventional IVF and do not show an increased risk of birth defects compared to the general population.

The major limitation of PGD for an older woman is that she needs to produce enough healthy embryos to make the procedure practical. Women age thirty-seven and older usually have a higher percentage of embryos harboring too few or too many chromosomes compared to younger women. We need a sufficient number of good-quality embryos to make an accurate genetic diagnosis and ensure we transfer normal embryos. In about 15 percent of couples undergoing PGD testing, no embryos are available for transfer.

One of the potential problems with genetic testing of a single cell is that it may not always represent the chromosomal makeup of its neighboring cells. This may be due to a phenomenon called mosaicism, whereby the adjoining cells in the same embryo may have a different chromosomal makeup. PGS is accurate in 90 percent of cases. Due to the 10 percent error rate, we recommend that all women who become pregnant following PGD or PGS undergo prenatal diagnosis with chorionic villus sampling (CVS) or amniocentesis.

Recently, newer technology using a method that assesses multiple sites on the chromosomes of DNA, called *single nucleotide polymorphisms* (SNPs), has made it possible to evaluate all twenty-three chromosome pairs simultaneously. Not all labs are capable of providing this service. When it is available, the embryo can be tested for specific gene defects at the same time.

It still remains to be seen whether PGD and PGS improve pregnancy rates in older women who do not get pregnant with IVF. It does seem to be very helpful for couples with recurrent miscarriages where there is a definite chromosomal abnormality in either parent. Testing the single cell in these instances allows the IVF team to transfer normal or chromosomally balanced embryos, resulting in reduction in miscarriage rates.

PGD adds about $3,000 to $6,000 to the cost of an IVF procedure, depending on the type of genetic analysis the couple requires.

Single-Gene Defects

More than two hundred single-gene defects can be detected with PGD. Theoretically, PGD can detect any alterations in DNA. Information is currently available for more than ten thousand genes, and that number continues to increase with advances in genetic technology.

One of the best characterized genes is one for cystic fibrosis, with more than one thousand mutations identified. Many of the mutations on this gene cause severe cystic fibrosis. PGD testing for these main mutations can potentially eliminate the risk of a couple having an affected child. We have worked out protocols to detect the main mutations in cystic fibrosis, and we get virtually instantaneous results. However, for a less frequent or newly discovered gene mutation, it may take a few weeks to several months to develop a new protocol in our PGD laboratory.

PGD for the evaluation of single-gene defects generally requires the DNA from the single cell of the embryo to be amplified through polymerase chain reaction (PCR). This biochemical technique makes millions of copies of the DNA in a matter of hours and provides enough DNA for genetic analysis.

Sophisticated methods utilizing DNA chip technology allow us to diagnose many genes simultaneously. The ability to DNA-fingerprint a single cell has made it possible to analyze a blastomere accurately after conventional IVF or ICSI.

PGD *Successes at* Weill *Cornell*

At Weill Cornell, we have been able to apply our research in PGD testing to help certain couples have disease-free babies. PGD has become a powerful diagnostic tool for couples who carry genetic traits that they do not wish to pass along to their children. It has been extremely exciting to see the fruits of years of research be so helpful to our patients. So far, with the use of PGD testing, we have helped four hundred couples to have healthy children.

Other Uses *of* PGD

Originally developed to identify the relatively small number of embryos at high risk for serious or fatal genetic diseases, PGD testing has expanded to encompass genetic tests for a growing number of illnesses, including some that are not necessarily fatal. Tests are already available for genetic variants associated with more than one thousand conditions, including deadly childhood illnesses, disorders linked to the X chromosome such as hemophilia, muscular dystrophy, and mental retardation, and adult-onset diseases such as Huntington disease and Alzheimer disease. More gene-specific diseases are being discovered as the technology advances.

PGD is also being used to evaluate gene mutations that might predispose a baby to certain types of cancer, for example, the targeted mutation *BRCA1* and *BRCA2* genes for hereditary breast cancer. Any daughter born with the *BRCA1* gene has an 80 percent risk of developing breast cancer and a 60 percent chance of developing ovarian cancer, as well as a 50 percent risk of passing on the genes to her own children.

However, this use of PGD testing is fraught with ethical issues. A child who does not carry the *BRCA1* gene has a reduced risk of breast cancer, but she could still get the disease. Other genes have been implicated in breast and ovarian cancer, but not as strongly as *BRCA1* and *BRCA2*.

A number of environmental factors, such as smoking, drinking too much alcohol, obesity, and diet, may also affect a woman's risk of developing breast cancer.

In addition, PGD testing allows parents to make choices about future children unrelated to their risks of serious childhood illnesses. For example, some parents have used PGD to attempt to have a baby who is an immunological match for an existing seriously ill child and then use the baby's umbilical-cord blood for stem-cell transplantation. This has been approved by several national oversight groups. Some couples have requested that PGD be used to help create a child with deafness or dwarfism so that they can have a child who shares their own condition. This is highly controversial since it can place that child at a great societal disadvantage.

One of the most controversial uses for PGD testing is to choose the sex of a child. Since this rarely has medical justification, some fertility clinics will not offer PGD solely for sex selection. In general, PGD has been used to eliminate the transmission of devastating sex-linked diseases in families who do not wish to transmit the abnormality to their offspring.

As more disease-linked gene variants are discovered, couples may face so many choices that it will be difficult to determine which genetic combination will produce the healthiest child. Surveys show that most people would elect to have prenatal genetic testing for life-altering conditions but not for enhancements such as athletic ability or superior intelligence. An international survey of 22,500 people shows that PGD is widely accepted for the purpose of selecting embryos that do not carry a defective gene or to cure a sibling suffering from some genetic disease, as well as to avoid embryos that carry a gene predisposing them to some grave adulthood disease, but not to choose the sex of a baby.

In the Future

Women over age thirty-seven who produce only a few normal embryos and have a diminishing number of eggs may benefit from methods to identify the best embryos to transfer or to choose the best eggs to fertilize in an IVF cycle and the best sperm to fertilize the eggs.

Identifying the Best Embryo for Transfer

Australian researchers at Monash University have developed a novel strategy of utilizing a combination of blastocyst biopsy, DNA fingerprinting, and genetic probes to identify the best embryos to transfer. Their ultimate aim is to find out which genes are expressed by the most viable embryos.

The researchers recruited forty-eight women undergoing IVF, retrieved and fertilized their eggs, and cultured the embryos for five days until they became blastocysts. They removed from eight to twenty cells from the blastocysts and analyzed the genes expressed in these cells. One or more blastocysts were transferred to all forty-eight women, and twenty-five became pregnant, with thirty-seven babies being born.

Blood from the umbilical cords or from swabs of cheek cells was taken from the babies and stored. The researchers used DNA fingerprinting on these samples to match them with the DNA obtained from the blastocyst biopsies. This allowed them to identify which embryo grew into which baby. Then they analyzed the genetic material to find out which genes were expressed in the viable blastocysts.

They have discovered that genes known to be involved in key processes in embryo implantation are expressed in the viable blastocysts. If we can further refine the set of genes involved, this process could be used to select the single most viable embryo for fertilization or transfer. This will likely take several years of research.

Other investigators have used protein (proteomics) or biochemical profiles (metabolomics) to identify good-quality embryos. This research is ongoing, but its usefulness has yet to be demonstrated.

Choosing the Best Eggs for IVF

Genetic clues contained in the cells that nurture developing eggs could help identify which ones to choose for IVF. When an egg is developing, it is nurtured by specialized cells called cumulus cells. These cells provide the nutrients the egg needs to grow. Researchers at the University of Lyon in France wondered whether there were genetic markers in these cells that could predict the quality of an embryo and the likelihood of a successful pregnancy.

They retrieved eggs and the cumulus cells from thirty women undergoing IVF. After freezing the cumulus cells, they fertilized the eggs via an ICSI procedure and inspected the quality of the resulting embryos. They then looked at the gene expression profiles of the cumulus cells corresponding to the eggs that produced good and bad embryos, as well as those that failed to fertilize.

Their analysis found that the expression of three genes was strongly associated with embryo quality. They plan to use the three genetic markers to select eggs, fertilize and implant them, and then see how many of these embryos yield healthy pregnancies as compared with embryos from unscreened eggs. It remains to be proven whether it will become a valuable tool to screen eggs.

Choosing the Best Sperm for IVF

Techniques have been developed that can identify sperm with healthy DNA and normal genes, but these techniques currently require the sperm to be fixed (killed), rendering them useless for ICSI. On the horizon are techniques that will not kill the sperm. Experiments in rats have successfully reversed aging effects by wiping out the testicular cells with a chemical and then allowing them to regenerate. The new cells are like young ones. However, rats are not humans, and this technique is years away from application to humans.

Take-Home Messages

- Various ovarian-stimulation strategies may improve your response to gonadotropins and enhance your chance of retrieving more eggs.
- Your AMH levels may help predict your response to ovarian stimulation.
- Co-culture of embryos with your own endometrial cells may improve your chances for IVF success, particularly if you have not become pregnant in previous IVF or ICSI attempts and have exhibited poor embryo quality.
- You may be a good candidate for assisted hatching if your embryos are thick-shelled or highly fragmented or several IVF attempts have failed.
- PGD tests provide information about the genetic status of your embryos to help ensure that only embryos that are free of problems are transferred. Tests are already available for genetic variants associated with more than one thousand medical conditions.

Thirteen

Third-Party Reproduction
Egg Donation, Embryo Donation, Sperm Donation, and Gestational Carrier

. . . .

"We had tried to get pregnant for quite awhile," says Janet, a forty-four-year-old city official. "My husband, Saul's, sperm count was very low because of a varico-cele. His sperm count improved somewhat after Dr. Goldstein fixed the varicocele through surgery, but it was still low, so he suggested we try direct sperm injection." Their first cycle of in vitro fertilization (IVF) with intracytoplasmic sperm injec-tion (ICSI) didn't work. "The hormone injections threw off the chemistry of my periods, even afterward," says Janet.

A second ICSI cycle was canceled because she developed only a single follicle. "Dr. Rosenwaks told me that because of my age and poor ovarian response, I was unlikely to become pregnant with my own eggs. He recommended egg dona-tion," says Janet. They chose an egg donor who had been recruited and specifically screened by the program at Weill Cornell. "She matched my looks, and I liked that she was from the same ethnic background as me," Janet says.

Janet and Saul, a fifty-six-year-old musician, met with a psychologist to dis-cuss their feelings on using an egg donor. "We talked about how the baby would not have my genetic material. I realized it didn't make a difference to me, and it didn't to Saul," Janet recalls. Once they signed the egg-donor consent forms, the egg donor was stimulated to produce eggs, and Janet's endometrial development *was synchronized with the donor's. "We had the option of sharing her eggs with another couple, but we did not take that option, and it was good that we didn't. She had very few good-quality eggs," Janet says. Four of the donor's eggs were inseminated with Saul's sperm, and two were transferred into Janet's uterus.*

A little less than nine months later, her twin boys were born. The two boys stayed in the hospital for three weeks. "The day we brought them home, I was so panicked," Janet recalls. "It's a lot of work being a mother of twins. I love my children."

. . . .

Even if you have had many frustrations in your journey to have a pregnancy— tests, doctor's visits, needles, and disappointment after disappointment—and have run through the gamut of fertility treatments, including IVF and ICSI, without success, you may still be able to have a baby with a donation of eggs, embryos, or sperm.

A donor-egg program is an alternative for women who are unable to use their own eggs to become pregnant. Even a few years ago, these women had no chance to experience pregnancy and childbirth. Today, using egg dona- tion procedures that were first pioneered in Australia and the United States by doctors presently at Weill Cornell, we are able to help many women experience childbirth and start a family. We perform about two hundred donor-egg transfers per year, and more than half of them result in live births.

With so many frozen embryos now stored in fertility clinics, a donor embryo program has become an option for many couples who can't have a child together. A frozen embryo from another couple is thawed and then transferred in a standard IVF cycle to allow a woman to bear a child.

In the not-too-distant past, donor sperm was one of the most popular and successful methods for treating severe male-factor problems. Now, with the advent of ICSI, we don't use sperm from a donor as often. There are still certain situations in which donor sperm is an option, particularly as a backup to sperm aspiration or an IVF procedure.

For each of the third-party reproductive options outlined in this chapter, we explore the social, ethical, and legal ramifications as well as the medical issues.

Egg Donation

If a woman is unable to produce a viable egg, then a donor egg becomes her primary option. This offers the opportunity for both partners to participate in the creation of their child—the man genetically through his sperm and the woman biologically through carrying the pregnancy.

An egg-donation program is most useful for a woman who has premature ovarian failure, that is, her ovaries lose their function before she reaches forty. Egg donation is also an option for a woman who has had her ovaries removed or has lost ovarian function due to cancer or cancer treatments and in rare cases to prevent transmission of a genetic disease.

Before a couple enters into a program to receive donated eggs, Dr. Rosenwaks evaluates both the woman and the man. He will evaluate the woman's uterine cavity using a hysterogram or a sonohysterogram to detect any abnormalities. He will also perform an ultrasound scan during the woman's cycle to assess the thickness of her endometrium, and if it is too thin, he will investigate the reason for this.

If she is over forty-five, he may also assess her heart function and her potential for pregnancy-induced hypertension or gestational diabetes, which could interfere with her carrying the pregnancy to term. With advancing age, a woman's uterus may become less receptive due to as-yet-undefined mechanisms as well as a higher likelihood of fibroid tumors, polyps, or uterine adhesions.

Her male partner provides a semen sample for analysis to decide whether he has enough healthy sperm to undergo an IVF cycle and, if not, whether an ICSI procedure will be required. The man also has any necessary genetic tests indicated by his ethnic background and receives treatment for any infectious diseases.

How to Select an Egg Donor

There are three ways to find an egg donor. The first is through an egg donor identified and recruited through an established program or egg-donor agency. The second approach is to ask your younger friends or relatives to see whether someone is willing to donate an egg. The third is through young women undergoing IVF at a fertility clinic who may agree to donate their excess eggs to infertile patients, which in some states is allowed only for altruistic reasons.

Whether the egg donor is anonymous or known, she must go through a screening process. This process takes into account the woman's age, height, weight, general health, family medical history, background, education, and lifestyle. In most cases, egg donors are between the ages of twenty-one and thirty-three, have a body mass index of less than 25 (that is, they are not overweight), are nonsmokers, have a high school diploma or college degree, and are able to pass physical and psychological screenings. Sometimes egg donor applicants are disqualified if they have a family history of diseases or if they were adopted and cannot provide a family medical history. In the United States, the Food and Drug Administration (FDA) requires that all egg donors be screened for risk factors and clinical evidence of communicable infections and diseases. Donors go through a battery of medical and psychological screenings to ensure that they are healthy and capable of making an informed decision to donate. Only about 12 percent of women who apply make it through the screening process at Weill Cornell.

Ideally, the prospective egg donor should be evaluated by a genetic counselor to identify any risk factors for genetic diseases. Prospective donors of all ethnic groups should be screened for the most common genetic diseases, for example, Mediterranean donors should be screened for beta-thalassemia, Southeast Asian and Chinese donors for alpha-thalassemia, donors of African descent for sickle cell anemia, and Ashkenazi Jewish donors for Tay-Sachs and Canavan disease and other Ashkenazi-prone genetic diseases. A complete genetic screening may include a chromosome analysis as well as testing for common genetically transmitted disorders such as fragile X syndrome and cystic fibrosis.

The egg donor should provide information about her sexual habits and exposure to drug use. Her blood should be tested for infection with syphilis, hepatitis B and C, and human immunodeficiency virus (HIV). A cervical culture should test for gonorrhea, mycoplasma, and chlamydia. These tests should be done at the initial screening and should be repeated during the egg retrieval cycle.

Some women who investigate the possibility of becoming an egg donor drop the idea once they learn what it entails. All told, it's a ninety- to 120-day commitment that has some health risks, although the risks are relatively low. In a study of nearly six hundred egg donors who had nearly nine hundred egg retrievals, we found that fewer than 1 percent of the egg donors had serious complications, including ovarian hyperstimulation syndrome (OHSS), twisted ovaries, infection, or ruptured ovarian cysts. With careful monitoring, the egg donors in the study experienced lower rates of OHSS than infertile women undergoing IVF. Minor complications, such as anesthesia reactions and bleeding into the abdomen or bladder, may occur but are easily controlled.

There are no long-term studies on the effects of egg donation on the donor's fertility. And there aren't likely to be any, because the process is generally anonymous in the United States. There is no registry of health information from women who've donated their eggs. The federal government's Centers for Disease Control is only required to ask fertility clinics how many successful births result from donor eggs.

Egg-Donor Procedure

Once a couple and donor have been matched, they sign the Weill Cornell consent forms. These forms lay out the potential physical and psychological risks for both the donor and the recipient couple. In addition, the egg donor and the recipient couple are informed of their obligations and rights.

The most important medical aspect of egg donation is the synchronization of the recipient's cycle with the egg donor's stimulation cycle. The donor cycle is programmed by either starting the donor on birth control pills—to control the day she begins her ovarian stimulation—or placing her on a gonadotropin-releasing hormone (GnRH) agonist to suppress her own cycle. The recipient's cycle is also suppressed with GnRH agonists, which are hormones that interfere with LH and FSH production.

Once the recipient's cycle is suppressed, she begins treatment with estradiol in skin patches, pills, or injections, followed by progesterone treatments either by injections or vaginally to prepare her endometrium. Normally, the endometrium is ready to receive a developing embryo for implantation between day 17 and day 19. Since the window of implantation is relatively short, Dr. Rosenwaks coordinates the development of the embryo with the progression of the recipient's endometrium. The recipient begins progesterone on the day after the donor receives human chorionic gonadotropin (hCG) or a GnRH agonist to induce ovulation.

When the donor starts her hormonal medications to stimulate her ovaries, the recipient is given estradiol to stimulate the endometrium to develop. Throughout the first phase of the egg-donation cycle, the egg donor gives herself a series of injections with ovulation-inducing drugs and makes frequent visits to the fertility clinic to monitor her ovulation through blood tests and ultrasound scans. She is asked either to abstain from sex completely or to use birth control to make sure she does not become pregnant.

During this time, the recipient takes increasing doses of estradiol. Dr. Rosenwaks may have to adjust the estradiol doses to synchronize her cycle with the egg donor's cycle. If the recipient has some ovarian function, he may need to use a GnRH agonist or GnRH antagonist to suppress her menstrual cycle temporarily.

To create the embryo, either the recipient's partner's sperm is mixed with the donor eggs to fertilize them for an IVF cycle, or a single sperm is injected into each of the donor eggs for an ICSI cycle. Three to five days later, one or two embryos are transferred to the recipient's uterus using the standard technique. Any extra embryos are frozen for future attempts to achieve a pregnancy.

After the embryo transfer, the recipient continues to take small doses of estradiol through the rest of her cycle. Dr. Rosenwaks continues the progesterone injections to help support the luteal phase of her cycle. If the recipient develops fever or an inflammatory reaction to the progesterone injections, he substitutes a progesterone vaginal suppository. If the woman becomes pregnant, she continues taking estradiol and progesterone through the first trimester to support the early pregnancy.

As with other ART procedures, the major risk of donor egg programs is multiple gestations, and that's why we now transfer only one or two embryos per cycle. Our multiple pregnancy rate is 30 percent to 40 percent, with most of these being twins. More recently, the trend has been to transfer a single embryo.

The cost of an egg donation may vary according to your geographic location. Insurance covers the medical procedures in some states, but not the donor fees.

Egg-Donor Compensation

Almost everyone who participates in egg donation agrees that the donor should be compensated for her time lost at work or school and the inconvenience and discomfort of the procedure. However, the amount of compensation varies, depending on the fertility clinic's policies, regional differences, and the involvement of agencies.

The procedure asks a lot of egg donors. They have to follow a strict schedule of injections and to go through some uncomfortable and sometimes painful procedures. Their compensation recognizes that egg donation requires serious dedication and effort.

Surveys of fertility clinics throughout the United States show that the average level of compensation provided for egg donors is less than $5,000. The ethics committee of the American Society for Reproductive Medicine (ASRM) advises that sums of more than $5,000 require justification, and compensation of more than $10,000 goes beyond what is appropriate. These guidelines explicitly state that compensation should be for the egg donor's time and commitment.

Nearly seventy egg-donor agencies have signed an agreement with the ASRM's Society for Assisted Reproductive Technology (SART) that they will abide by the ASRM ethics committee guidelines governing payments to donors (available at http://www.asrm.org/Patients/eggdonor_agencies .pdf). An agency typically charges a fee of slightly more than $4,000 for its services, which include locating a donor for a couple. However, these agencies may not necessarily comply with the ASRM guidelines on compensation. Some agencies ask for premium fees for donors with preferred qualifications, while others charge more than $10,000 for egg-donor compensation.

Some young women donate eggs to help relatives and friends or from a sense of altruism, but others openly acknowledge that money is a big factor in their decision. Surveys show that most egg donors use their compensation to pay off credit-card debt and other loans or for everything from savings and downpayments on property to school expenses and car payments. Studies show the women who donate eggs primarily for altruistic reasons feel happier about their donation experience than do women who donate mainly for the money.

"Egg Donors Wanted" ads are common on the Internet, in college newspapers, and on trains and buses. Eggs have become a commodity. With no federal laws limiting donor fees, policing the egg-donor market is very difficult, if not impossible. The usual fee for egg donation is determined geographically. Most clinics steer away from excessive fees that could lead to coercion and affect the donor's decisions.

Embryo Donation

An estimated half-million frozen embryos sit in storage facilities in fertility clinics across the United States. When a couple decide that their family is complete, yet their frozen embryos are still available, they face the dilemma of what to do with them: discard them, donate them to research, or donate them to a couple who is unable to conceive. Most couples who undergo IVF plan to use their frozen embryos for future pregnancies. On an emotional level, they think of them as potential babies. But a couple might decide not to have any more children, their marriage might dissolve, or a spouse might die. The couple or survivor must decide whether to pay the annual cost of keeping the embryos frozen.

Embryo donation may be indicated for a couple that is unable to conceive, either naturally or with assisted reproduction techniques, a couple with genetic disorders affecting one or both partners, or a single woman who has untreatable infertility.

The decision to donate embryos—to allow someone else to have babies that bear your genes—is often difficult. Weill Cornell counselors are available to help potential embryo donors work through the decision-making process. Once they decide to donate, the embryo donors sign a consent agreement that signs over ownership of the embryos to the Weill Cornell fertility clinic.

The potential recipient couple sort through the histories of donors who are willing to donate their leftover embryos. The recipient couple receive some basic information about the donor couple: their education, physical characteristics (height and weight), ethnic background, and medical history. This allows the couple to select embryos with a likelihood of having the characteristics they desire in a child. The identity of the donor remains anonymous.

Before agreeing to an embryo donation, a couple should make sure the embryo donors have had a medical and genetic workup. At least six months after the embryos have been frozen, the donor couple should be tested for HIV, hepatitis B and C, and syphilis. The donor couple should have appropriate genetic screening, if it has not already been done.

Egg donation and embryo donation are both under Food and Drug Administration (FDA) regulation. Each fertility clinic may set its own limits but must comply with FDA and state regulations. In addition, some clinics allow the donating couple to meet the recipient couple, which is a common practice among adoption agencies when a child is adopted. Some clinics also require a "home study" of the recipient couple.

Once the consent forms have been signed and the embryos for donation have been identified, the embryos are thawed and transferred to the recipient woman using the same synchronization scheme and estrogen and progesterone replacement described for egg donation recipients. The recipient woman faces all of the typical risks of pregnancy as well as the increased risks of multiple pregnancy if two or more embryos are transferred at the same time. Many couples insist that more than one embryo be transferred to increase their chances of having a child.

One of the aspects that makes embryo donation appealing is the relatively low cost, which is about $5,000. This is considerably less than repeated IVF or ICSI attempts or the adoption of a child. An embryo donation is usually quick, taking between six and twelve months to complete successfully. Success rates with embryo donation depend on the quality of the embryos that were frozen, the age of the woman who provided the eggs, and the number of embryos transferred.

Embryo donation can be controversial for both ethical and legal reasons. A child born to the recipient couple has no genetic link to them. This differs from egg or sperm donation, where one partner provides half of the child's genes. The embryo donors and the recipient couple should receive counseling to address all the potential issues and concerns they may have. Also, because there are no laws that deal explicitly with embryo donation and regulations vary from state to state, the couples should consult with attorneys to see whether they need a predonation legal agreement with the genetic parents.

Gestational Carrier

A gestational carrier is a woman who carries a pregnancy for a couple who have created an embryo with their own sperm and eggs or from donor sperm or a donor egg. This is different from a surrogate mother, who is a woman who carries a pregnancy for another couple with an embryo created with her own egg and the sperm of the infertile couple's male partner or their chosen sperm donor.

Typically, the couple undergo an IVF procedure to produce a number of embryos. One or more embryos will then be placed in the uterus of the gestational carrier, who carries the baby to term. When the child is born, the carrier will turn the baby over to the couple and sign away her parental rights.

A gestational carrier may be the best fertility solution for a woman who has normally functioning ovaries but lacks a uterus. Others who may benefit are women who can't risk a pregnancy because of a health problem such as severe heart disease, systemic lupus erythematosis, a history of breast cancer, severe kidney disease, cystic fibrosis, severe diabetes mellitus, or a history of severe high blood pressure during pregnancy, or because of an abnormally shaped uterus with a history of repeated miscarriages.

There are two ways to identify a gestational carrier. The first is to find a friend or relative to volunteer to carry your pregnancy. The second is to identify a woman through an agency that recruits potential carriers. Ideally, the carrier should be under age thirty, have delivered a live baby after a full-term pregnancy, and have a history of pregnancies without complications.

Once a couple identifies a gestational carrier, an obstetrician evaluates her overall health and screens her for underlying medical conditions that might complicate a pregnancy. This includes a detailed history of her pregnancies, births, and lifestyle and a physical examination. The doctor evaluates her uterine cavity with a hysterosalpingogram, sonohysterogram, or hysteroscopy.

The couple also undergoes a complete medical history and physical examination. The man has a semen analysis and the woman has an evaluation of her ovarian function. Both partners are screened for infectious diseases, including syphilis, gonorrhea, chlamydia, cytomegalovirus (CMV), HIV, and hepatitis B and C. The carrier is screened for the same infectious diseases, as well as immunity to rubella, rubeola, and varicella.

A counselor makes sure the carrier understands the potential risks of becoming pregnant and helps the carrier and her partner, if she has one, explore this emotionally intense arrangement. This includes how to manage their relationship with the parents-to-be, how to cope with feelings of attachment to the fetus during the pregnancy, and how carrying a baby will impact their children, friends, family members, and employers.

In addition, the carrier and parents-to-be should discuss their ongoing relationship with the counselor. In particular, they should discuss the number of embryos to be transferred, prenatal diagnosis, and what to do if there is a multiple pregnancy or if the pregnancy needs to be terminated because the fetus has a severe defect.

Gestational-carrier arrangements are usually set up by contracts arranged through an agency or as independent adoptions in states where this is legal. The couple usually pays the carrier's expenses, including doctor's visits, housing, and the legal, agency, and service fees, as specified by the contract.

The compensation for the carrier varies depending on state laws. Most states do not allow the carrier to be compensated. Others permit a court to issue an order of parentage before the birth, which allows the couple to be listed as parents on the birth certificate without an adoption; these orders legally allow carrier compensation. In states where compensation is legal, the contract for a carrier through an agency can cost more than $50,000, with about $25,000 going to the carrier and $15,000 or more to the agency, plus insurance and legal expenses.

Insurance companies have become more aware of the costs of a gestational carrier, and some companies have added exclusions to policies for any kind of surrogate birth. If you use a gestational carrier, have a reproductive lawyer check the fine print in the carrier's insurance policy to rule out this type of exclusion.

The legal aspects of using a gestational carrier can be complex. Intricate contracts and arrangements are often required to ensure that the procedure is successful for both the carrier and the parents-to-be. Legal counsel is essential before entering into an agreement with a woman who will serve as a gestational carrier.

Sperm Donation

The frequency of artificial insemination of donor sperm has changed dramatically, thanks to the introduction of ICSI. Even when a man has a very low sperm count or low motility, or no sperm at all in the ejaculate, doctors can isolate a single sperm from the ejaculate or retrieve sperm from the testicles to inject directly into an egg. We may use donor sperm if a man has a zero sperm count (azoospermia) and we fail to identify any sperm surgically. Sperm donation is rarely used to overcome genetic disorders. Nowadays we perform preimplantation genetic diagnosis (PGD) on embryos when either or both partners carry a significant genetic defect.

A single woman without a male partner may also use donor sperm.

Sperm donation is always an option for a couple going through an IVF cycle. In general, to avoid canceling an IVF cycle, Dr. Rosenwaks will offer the couple donor sperm as a backup on the day of egg retrieval in case the man's sperm is not available or viable.

To choose a sperm donor, most fertility clinics refer couples to counselors affiliated with individual sperm banks. The sperm-bank counselor guides the couple through the process of selecting a sperm donor. Couples try to choose a donor who resembles the man, based on age, education, occupation, religion, ethnicity, and physical characteristics, including height and weight, eye and hair color, and blood type. You can also choose a friend or relative to donate sperm.

Since the emergence of AIDS in the 1980s, donor insemination has been performed exclusively with frozen sperm. FDA and ASRM guidelines recommend that sperm be quarantined for at least six months before being used in donor inseminations. The sperm donor must fill out a comprehensive medical questionnaire to evaluate his health and review his family medical history. He is tested for syphilis, chlamydia, gonorrhea, HIV, CMV, and hepatitis B and C. FDA regulations require that his sperm be free of infectious diseases within seven days of all donations and that the sperm be tested every six months as long as he is a donor. If you choose a known donor, he should have the same screening as an anonymous donor, and both the donor and recipient must undergo extensive counseling and psychological evaluations.

The sperm from the donor must meet minimum standards, usually 20 to 30 million moving sperm per milliliter after thawing, with 25 percent to 40 percent sperm motility. Sperm banks keep the frozen donated sperm in divided portions or vials. In general, the bank sends us two to four vials of donor sperm for each couple. We save the leftover donor sperm for another cycle, if necessary. We also recommend that couples reserve additional samples from the same sperm donor at the sperm bank. This allows the couple's child to have a biologically related sibling at some time in the future.

The cost of a donor sperm sample is about $150. Most insurance companies do not reimburse for donated sperm.

Before the donor insemination, we document the woman's ovulation either with an ovulation predictor kit or with daily blood tests at mid-cycle. When necessary, a hysterogram is performed to evaluate the uterine cavity and whether the fallopian tubes are open before insemination. The donor insemination can either be timed to a natural cycle or be part of an ovulation induction cycle.

The simple insemination procedure takes place close to the time of ovulation. Dr. Rosenwaks draws up the thawed semen sample into a catheter, inserts the catheter into the woman's cervix, and usually injects the sperm into the uterus. If he suspects the woman may have a reproductive tract infection, then he performs a cervical or vaginal insemination. If the couple require an intrauterine insemination, for example, due to hostile cervical mucus, then a washed semen sample is placed through the cervix and into her uterus.

The success of donor insemination depends on the woman's age and whether she has any other female infertility factors, including endometriosis, fallopian tube disease, or ovulation problems. Pregnancy rates per cycle range from 8 percent to 15 percent, with higher success with IUI than with simple artificial insemination. The risk of birth defects is no higher with a child conceived through donor insemination than from a natural conception.

A sperm donor is usually compensated about $100 for every acceptable donation, but it's not easy money. It's not like in the movies, where a man shows up, makes a deposit, and gets handed a check. The sperm-donor screening process requires that the man be at least 5 feet 9 inches, eighteen to thirty-eight years old, live near the sperm bank, have a college degree or be enrolled in a four-year university, be in good health, be free of sexual diseases, have a high sperm yield, and submit a family medical history. Less than 10 percent of applicants are accepted as sperm donors. Once accepted, a man must agree to make one to three deposits weekly for twelve to eighteen months. There is a financial incentive, but most sperm donors have an altruistic side as well, hoping to help an infertile couple to have a baby.

Before using donor sperm, we strongly suggest the couple seek the support and guidance of one of our psychologists who specialize in infertility. Men who feel strongly about their family history may feel that donor sperm severs these ties. These men must face their sadness about not being able to see some of their own traits reflected in their children. Both the man and the woman must learn to accept that the child they are about to create is indeed their own.

Couples who can't produce a child related to both partners have to come to terms with this loss of ability to procreate a genetic offspring. They may feel sad, angry, or grief-stricken and may lose their hopes, self-esteem, and even their health. Either partner may experience these feelings, regardless of whose fertility is lost. A counselor can help the couple explore their feelings and lead them toward accepting egg, embryo, or sperm donation as a way to build a family.

At Weill Cornell, we require that all individuals wishing to use sperm or egg donation be counseled by our highly trained psychologists. This is both to ensure proper awareness of the process and to review the psychological, social, and emotional aspects of gamete donation.

In the Future

Studies are ongoing to develop genetic markers that will identify women who are likely to develop premature ovarian failure and consequently may become infertile prematurely. Other genetic markers that may be associated with infertility are being investigated. For example, our own studies have identified genetic variations in the progesterone receptor and a tumor-suppressor gene called p53. Although these are early studies, they point out that the application of genetic screening will allow us to define new causes of infertility.

Several groups, including our own, are investigating the possibility of generating new germ cells—eggs and sperm—from a woman's or man's body (somatic) cells. When this becomes possible, it could revolutionize and possible eliminate infertility.

Genetic Links to Premature Ovarian Failure

In looking for genes that cause premature ovarian failure, Baylor University researchers are concentrating on mutations they believe might accelerate the loss of eggs. They have screened a hundred women and found three different kinds of mutations in the genes that control early egg development.

In their ongoing studies, they hope to define the majority of the genes in the pathways involved in ovarian failure and find biomarkers in the blood that can help determine a woman's risk of early infertility. Ideally, they will be able to offer a test that looks at all of the genes involved in premature ovarian failure, but that type of test will take years of research.

Researchers in the Netherlands have studied the genes of more than ten thousand women who had gone through menopause and have found a connection between slightly earlier menopause and twenty common genetic variants on two chromosomes. They intend to study the exact biology and effect of this association to get a better understanding of the function of these genetic variants in early menopause.

Take-Home Messages

- You may be a good candidate for egg donation if you have failed many IVF cycles and are over age forty, have failed with IVF due to poor embryo quality, have premature ovarian failure, your ovaries have been removed, or you have lost ovarian function due to cancer.
- Prospective egg donors, whether anonymous or known to you, must go through a rigorous psychological, medical, and genetic screening process.
- To perform the egg-donation procedure, the egg donor's menstrual cycle must become synchronized with the egg recipient's cycle.
- The amount you compensate an egg donor depends on the fertility clinic's policies, regional differences, and the involvement of egg-donation agencies.
- Embryo donation may be a good fertility choice if you have been unable to conceive either naturally or with assisted reproduction techniques, you have genetic disorders that affect either one or both partners and PGD cannot be successfully applied, or you are a single woman who has untreatable infertility.
- A gestational carrier may be the best fertility solution if you have normally functioning ovaries but lack a uterus. You may also benefit if you can't risk a pregnancy because of a health problem or you have an abnormally shaped uterus that cannot be surgically corrected and a history of repeat miscarriages.
- Donor sperm may be a potential option if you have a zero sperm count and you have no sperm that can be identified surgically, or you are a single woman without a male partner.

Fourteen

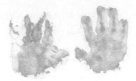

Other Fertility Issues
The Potential of Stem Cells

· · · · · · · · · ·

"When we began planning for an in vitro fertilization (IVF) procedure, Bob and I didn't think much about what we'd do if we had any extra embryos. All we wanted was enough viable embryos to have a baby," recalls Karen, a forty-year-old sociologist. She and Bob, a fifty-four-year-old businessman, had tried to start their family when she was thirty and he was forty-four. After several years with no success, each had a workup at Weill Cornell, and it was discovered that Bob's low sperm count required them to use IVF.

In their first IVF cycle, Bob and Karen froze six viable embryos and donated twelve non-viable embryos to research. "We didn't agonize much about the decision to donate. The doctors told us there was little chance those embryos would develop. We also believe in stem-cell research and thought that rather than our viable frozen embryos being destroyed, they should be donated to stem-cell research," says Karen.

Their first and second IVF attempts failed, but during their third try, three embryos were transferred, and one took. Their daughter, Alice, is now eight years old.

· · · · · · · · · ·

After more than one decade of painstaking stem-cell research, there are now promising results with both embryonic and adult stem cells. Stem cells are the master cells that can grow into every cell, tissue, and organ in the body. Scientists study them to understand the biology not only of disease, but of life itself. They want to use stem cells to transform medicine and find cures for such debilitating illnesses as Parkinson disease, heart disease, cancer, diabetes, and infertility. The theory behind this field, known as regenerative medicine, is that stem cells may one day be able to provide tissues to replace worn-out organs or nonfunctioning cells. Stem cells have the unique property of being able to multiply almost endlessly and transform themselves into almost any other type of cell. Scientists would like to devise ways to coax stem cells in the laboratory to become cells of various tissues, like the heart, the liver, or the pancreas, that can be injected into the organs to support the organs' function. Scientists also hope stem cells can be used to create new sperm or eggs to treat infertility.

There are two basic types of stem cells: embryonic stem cells and adult stem cells. Embryonic stem cells come from early embryos. They are usually isolated from surplus embryos created through IVF. Each cell from the early embryo has the power to become any of the many different cell and tissue types in the body.

Adult stem cells can be found at all times in the life of a person and they, too, can be directed toward developing different kinds of adult cells. Recently, scientists have discovered how to transform adult cells back to their original, unspecialized state so that they, too, have properties of stem cells. These stem cells are called induced pluripotent stem cells.

Federal Regulations

Stem cells have been surrounded by controversy for the past decade because they have primarily been collected from early-stage embryos. Shortly after President George W. Bush took office in 2001, he limited federal research spending to stem-cell lines then in existence. In August 2001, only about two dozen embryonic-stem-cell lines were made eligible for federal research funding. Most scientists now agree that these eligible lines are of limited use. Congress twice passed bills to allow potentially thousands more lines from surplus embryos to be used, but President Bush vetoed the bills. In the meantime, hundreds of stem-cell lines were created around the world from surplus embryos.

In April 2009, President Barack Obama lifted the ban by allowing federal funding for research on stem-cell lines created from surplus embryos at fertility clinics. The National Institutes of Health (NIH) drafted guideline proposals to allow scientists who receive federal funding to conduct research on future embryonic-stem-cell lines and on some of those hundreds of lines already created from surplus embryos in privately funded clinics.

The guidelines maintain the Bush administration's policy of denying funding for research that uses human embryos created for purposes of research. Scientists will still be allowed to do research on new stem-cell lines grown in privately financed laboratories or those not financed by the federal government. For example, many scientists receive research money from California's $3 billion stem-cell initiative, which runs through 2014. President Obama made it clear that scientists should not be allowed to clone embryos for human reproduction.

The NIH guidelines also tighten the consent requirements for the use of surplus embryos. If couples who have completed their families want to donate embryos, they must first be informed of all of their options, including disposing of the embryos. They must sign specific written consent forms to donate the embryos for research and they must be allowed to withdraw their consent up until the time the embryos are used for research. With the expansion of federal funding opportunities for embryonic-stem-cell research, we believe that more couples will become interested in donating their embryos for research after completing their families.

Just after President Obama's inauguration, the Food and Drug Administration approved the first human tests on embryonic stem cells. In this landmark study, researchers will inject embryonic stem cells into the spinal cord of eight to ten people who have recently suffered severe spinal-cord injuries. NIH has since approved thirty other embryonic stem cell research projects and it also has approved forty embryonic stem cell lines for use by researchers with federal funding, with about one hundred additional lines still pending review.

Adult Stem Cells

For many years, scientists tried to develop ways to extract stem cells from adult tissue to sidestep the ethical objections of doing research on embryonic stem cells. Adult stem cells can be found in blood, bone marrow, and various tissues. But these cells have become partly differentiated, meaning they are on their way to becoming individualized tissues and are not as flexible as embryonic cells.

In tests with mice, scientists devised alternative ways to produce stem cells without destroying embryos. Then several teams of scientists discovered how to reprogram ordinary human adult skin and connective tissue cells to behave like embryonic stem cells. And human blood cells have also been reprogrammed, providing researchers with several easily accessible, plentiful sources of stem cells.

In 2007, two groups of scientists, one at the University of Wisconsin and the other at Kyoto University in Japan, created stem cells through a method called cell reprogramming. The new method used viruses to insert programmed genes into adult cells to transform them into embryo-like ones. The cells they developed were termed *induced pluripotent stem cells.* "Pluripotent" means the cells have the ability to become any of the body's cell types, which could potentially provide doctors with the ability to re pair damaged tissues throughout the body. However, there was a major drawback—the viruses incorporated themselves into the cells' DNA at random places and could potentially cause mutations and cancers.

Other researchers began to offer evidence that induced pluripotent stem cells do in fact have potential to be medically useful. Using reprogrammed cells, researchers at the Whitehead Institute for Biomedical Research in Massachusetts successfully treated sickle cell anemia and relieved Parkinson disease symptoms in rats. They followed that with a big breakthrough—they developed a method of producing stem cells free of harmful reprogramming genes from human skin cells of Parkinson disease patients. The Whitehead scientists used the induced pluripotent stem cells to create dopamine-producing neurons, the type of cells that degenerate in Parkinson disease patients.

Soon after, researchers at the Scripps Research Institute in La Jolla, California, generated embryo-like stem cells from fibroblasts—cells that give rise to connective tissue—without using any genetic material. The Scripps scientists found that the reprogrammed stem cells from fibroblasts behaved indistinguishably from classic embryonic stem cells, including differentiating into various cell types such as heart muscle, nerve, and pancreatic cells.

These new techniques solved one of the most challenging safety hurdles associated with personalized stem-cell-based medicine. For the first time, scientists could make stem cells in the laboratory from adult cells without genetically altering them. These new cells also had a huge advantage over embryonic stem cells. These stem cells could be derived from the person's own cells, so cells or tissue made from those stem cells would not be rejected by their immune system.

Human blood may be another source of stem cells. Stem cells from the bone marrow turn into blood cells, but they can also become cells of virtually any tissue of the body. And they do so every day of our lives. Stem cells from the bone marrow are a natural source of renewal. Anytime you become injured, a signal is sent to the bone marrow to release stem cells. The stem cells travel through the blood and into the affected tissue. Once they arrive in the tissue, the stem cells multiply and slowly transform to repair the damage by becoming cells of that tissue.

Human blood can also morph into stem cells. Howard Hughes Medical Institute researchers have reprogrammed blood cells to act as embryonic stem cells. The researchers collected blood from a male donor and isolated a type of stem cell that produces only blood cells. These stem cells were cultured in growth factors and infected with viruses carrying genes normally expressed in embryonic stem cells. This reset the blood cells to an embryonic state. Further tests confirmed that the reprogrammed cells had become induced pluripotent stem cells.

Programmable cells generated from the blood are much easier to obtain and analyze than embryonic stem cells. Their use should enhance the pace of laboratory research into stem cells and help determine the therapeutic potential of induced pluripotent stem cells.

Scientists at Weill Cornell have extracted stem cells from seminiferous tubules (sperm-forming tubes) and coaxed them to produce a variety of tissues, including heart, muscle, and skin cells. We hope that human testicles will have the same potential to provide stem cells that can be used to replace a wide variety of human tissues, including even sperm.

Scientific research into embryonic and adult stem cells will probably move in tandem. To coax stem cells to grow new tissue, scientists need stem cells of all kinds, including from embryos, adult cells, the umbilical cord, and the bone marrow. Stem cell researchers believe that a wide variety of stem-cell sources will eventually allow them to treat as many diseases as possible.

Fertility Research

The success of intracytoplasmic sperm injection (ICSI) has stimulated researchers to expand their search for ways to overcome infertility. Part of that quest has been the attempt to replicate sperm and eggs through embryonic stem cells.

Scarcity of sperm due to poor sperm production still hinders the success of assisted reproductive technologies. Sperm generated in the laboratory could provide an alternative. The impetus to duplicate the genetic material in sperm was designed to study the underlying causes of male infertility. Weill Cornell researchers have extended this idea to replicate the genome of a mouse sperm cell and produce embryos capable of developing fully into newborn mice.

In one Weill Cornell experiment, researchers fused newly created sperm-like cells into two hundred mouse eggs. A total of 155 eggs began to divide, the first step in fertilization. Nearly all of the eggs grew into early embryos. During four days in a culture medium, about three quarters of them developed into blastocysts, which is comparable to the 80 percent of ICSI embryos that reach the blastocyst stage in our fertility patients. However, after transfer, 25 percent of the blastocysts developed into newborn mouse pups.

Production of cells derived from embryonic stem cells that will become an egg or sperm is another area of intense research. Stanford University researchers have used human embryos to create new cells that they hope eventually to manipulate into becoming eggs and sperm. In the laboratory, they have turned stem cells into cells that give rise to eggs and sperm. They are still working on how to supplement these cells so that they become capable of making embryos. It's unclear how long it will take for these experimental efforts to become a clinical reality.

Studies at Weill Cornell are ongoing in efforts to generate new eggs and sperm from mature cells. This may involve genetic reprogramming or even nuclear transfer technology, which involves transferring the complete genetic material from the nucleus of a cultured donor cell to a mature recipient egg whose own nucleus has been removed.

Sperm Developments

In the not-too-distant future, it may be possible for a man to be cured of disease through a biopsy of his own testicles. A new type of stem cell derived from a man's testicles could be useful for growing personalized replacement tissues such as heart muscle, blood vessels, and cartilage to help him fight disease and also overcome infertility. These stem cells are quite plentiful and natural, which gets around the need for embryonic stem cells. Stem cells from the sperm-producing testicles of men are very close in their development to the cells of embryos. So it's not too surprising that they would also prove extremely versatile in their ability to morph into many different types of tissue.

In 2007, Weill Cornell researchers used stem cells obtained from the testicles of mice and redirected the cells' development in the laboratory. The cells developed into working blood-vessel cells and tissue, as well as heart, nerve, and muscle cells. Unlike induced pluripotent stem cells, these mouse stem cells did not require any addition or tweaking of genes to get them to turn into these cell types.

These unique, specialized, early sperm-forming cells could be an easily accessible source of stem cells with exactly the same capability to form new tissues as embryonic stem cells have. The sole function of these cells is to generate the precursors to sperm. Normally, they are committed to that function only, and that's what keeps a man fertile as he ages. In their experiments, the Weill Cornell researchers concocted a biochemical environment for the cells that included particular helper-cell types and growth factors aimed at fostering the cells' development away from becoming sperm cells and toward developing into many different cell types.

Recently, a team at the University of Tübingen in Germany and researchers at Georgetown University and Stanford proved that this concept could work in humans. They extracted stem cells from the testicles of men who were fertility patients, organ donors, or undergoing medical treatment. The researchers found that after a few weeks of growth, these stem cells could differentiate into various types of cells, just like those taken from embryos.

These developments provide scientists with yet another source of stem cells. The next step is to get these differentiated cells to cure disease in animal models. Researchers are now testing whether sperm stem cells that have morphed into pancreatic cells can treat diabetes in mice.

The promise for men is that there may be a readily available source of stem cells that, once they are produced, can be frozen and used at any point in the future. These sperm-derived stem cells also avoid issues linked to tissue transplant rejection, since the stem cells come from the man's own body. What's more, the procedure could provide sperm for men who become infertile due to chemotherapy or radiation treatments.

Ethical Concerns

Many infertility patients see donating their remaining embryos for medical research as preferable to discarding them or to donating them to another infertile couple. A survey by Duke University and Johns Hopkins University researchers of more than two thousand couples who had frozen embryos in storage found that 60 percent said they would be more likely to donate the embryos for stem-cell research rather than discard them, donate them to other infertile couples, or store them indefinitely. About 40 percent of our IVF couples with extra embryos decide to donate them to research.

An online IVF ethics questionnaire conducted by Reproductive Biology Associates has established a positive view of stem-cell research in people around the world. More than six hundred members of the general public, IVF patients, doctors, and scientists working in the fertility field responded to the survey over a period of six weeks. On the two questions that dealt with embryonic stem cells, the vast majority thought it was not morally wrong to use embryonic stem cells for research or medical treatment. Despite media reports that people appear to be evenly split for and against the use of stem cells, this study shows that public, private, and scientific opinion is very much in favor of both stem-cell research and the therapeutic use of stem cells in medical treatment.

In the Future

For years, researchers have believed that a woman lost the capability to produce more eggs after she was born. However, actively dividing egg forming cells have been discovered in the ovaries of both young and adult mice. It's unclear whether these stem cells can regenerate eggs in women.

Stem Cells Spur New Eggs in Adult Mice

Could doctors someday use stem cells to help adult women produce brand-new eggs? This would run counter to the long-held belief that women are born with a finite number of eggs capable of being fertilized and becoming babies. Chinese researchers at Shanghai Jiao Tong University used stem cells from egg-making cells in mice, transformed them into eggs, and then transplanted them into infertile female mice, which were then able to produce offspring. If this can be performed in humans, it could offer the ability to generate new eggs in cases of female infertility or premature ovarian failure.

The Chinese researchers isolated active stem cells from the cells that normally give rise to eggs in female adult and five-day-old mice. They claim to have been able to generate new lines of these stem cells that proliferated even after being cultured multiple times. These stem cells restored fertility by producing new eggs when transplanted into the ovaries of female mice that had been rendered infertile by chemotherapy. The females then gave birth to normal mice.

This could be very exciting research, but there are many steps needed before this comes to fruition in humans. Even if the breakthrough could be applied to humans, it would likely be most useful to younger women with diminished ovarian reserves or those who are going through premature menopause.

Take-Home Messages

- Both embryonic and adult stem cells may be genetically transformed to become almost any tissue in the body.
- The latest guidelines expand opportunities for researchers to receive federal funding for embryonic-stem-cell research.
- Research on stem cells from embryos, adult cells, the umbilical cord, and bone marrow may allow researchers to develop treatments for many diseases.
- Scientists are working on how to replicate sperm and eggs using stem cells.
- Stem cells derived from a man's own testicles may become a readily available source of personalized tissues.

Fifteen

Can We Still Get Pregnant after Cancer?

Preserving Fertility after Diagnosis and Treatment

· · · · · · · · · ·

"We went to Weill Cornell for in vitro fertilization (IVF). It probably saved my life," says Tom, a fifty-three-year-old engineer. "I had a large varicocele on the left side and I had had surgery when I was about twelve for an undescended testicle on my right side. The two combined contributed to my low sperm count."

Dr. Goldstein surgically repaired his varicocele and asked him to follow up with yearly ultrasound scans of both testicles because men with a history of an undescended testicle are at risk of testicular cancer. "The next year, my wife, Tina, became pregnant with twins through IVF with direct sperm injection, and one month later I had my first sonogram of my scrotum. It showed I had testicular cancer," says Tom. "Dr. Goldstein told me it was the smallest tumor he had ever seen, and because it had been detected so early, it had not spread yet."

Three days after the discovery, Tom had outpatient surgery to remove the tiny testicular tumor, had sperm aspirated for future use, and then had radiation treatments for three weeks. "The surgery was easy, but the radiation was hard. I was tired a lot. The nausea was not so bad because I took pills continuously to prevent that," says Tom.

He was back to his old self quickly after the therapies. Now it's five years since he had the treatments. "I have no reason for concern. Basically, I'm cured," Tom says. "Because an undescended testicle is a risk factor for testicular cancer, I keep going for my yearly sonograms."

· · · · · · · · · ·

Cancer treatments such as chemotherapy and radiation can cause a woman to experience premature menopause and diminish her chance of getting pregnant. Similarly, chemotherapy, radiotherapy, or radical pelvic surgery can reduce a man's ability to produce sperm. Some 140,000 men and women younger than forty-five years old face a cancer diagnosis each year, but all is not lost for those who suffer from infertility caused by cancer treatments. Many survive treatment and are still young enough to have children.

Chemotherapy usually affects all body cells, attacking not only the cancer, but other tissues, including the ovaries and testicles. Unlike men, who produce sperm throughout their lifetime, women have only a set number of eggs from birth, and that number decreases as they age. Even young girls who undergo aggressive chemotherapy treatments often experience a sharp drop in the number of eggs, and some become completely sterile. Cancer treatments designed to kill fast-growing cancer cells may also affect rapidly dividing sperm-making cells. Sperm could be likened to the body's canary in a coal mine for toxic exposures, including radiation and chemotherapy, which quickly kill off sperm. Cancer cells are the most rapidly dividing cells, but sperm-making cells are the most rapidly dividing normal cells in the human body.

There are ways to preserve a woman's fertility, including freezing embryos, eggs, or tissue from her ovaries before she goes for cancer treatment. In the first and most effective method, a woman can undergo ovarian stimulation. The retrieved eggs are fertilized with her partner's or donor sperm. The newly created embryos are then frozen in anticipation that she will have the embryos placed in her uterus when she is cured. The second method is to retrieve her eggs and freeze them for thawing and fertilization later. This approach is most suitable for single women who do not want to use a sperm donor. In the third method, the outer layer of the ovary is removed, then frozen and preserved for later transplantation after the woman's treatment. For men, sperm collected before cancer treatment can be saved for many years. World-renowned cyclist Lance Armstrong has become a father for the fourth time after his sperm were preserved before his treatment for testicular cancer.

Strategies introduced in the late 1980s for protecting fertility in patients undergoing cancer treatment have helped boost reproduction rates among cancer survivors. However, female cancer survivors remain about half as likely as women who had never been diagnosed with the disease to have a child within the ten years following their diagnosis. For male cancer survivors, reproduction rates are about 30 percent lower than those of their healthy peers.

Cancer in Women

Not all women who are having cancer treatment have the opportunity to talk with a fertility specialist before beginning treatment. Yet there are several options for protecting the ovaries from chemotherapy and radiation therapy. Women who have been diagnosed with cancer may want to have some of their ovarian tissue or eggs collected and frozen in order to give them an opportunity to have children once their cancer treatment has finished.

Chemotherapy

. . . .

Margaret, a thirty-seven-year-old nurse, was diagnosed with stage II breast cancer. "My oncologist told me I would require chemotherapy after surgery. He said it was important for me to freeze my eggs or embryos before I had chemotherapy, since there was a chance I would lose my ability to have children," says Margaret. Although she wasn't married, Margaret discussed this with her fiancé, Allen. "Egg freezing was too risky, so we decided to go with IVF to create embryos and then freeze them in case I ended up with ovarian failure after my chemotherapy treatments," she says.

Margaret underwent a novel stimulation protocol developed at Weill Cornell using 5 milligrams per day of letrozole in conjunction with follicle-stimulating hormone (FSH). The stimulation was successful. Eight of her eggs were retrieved, and seven of the eight eggs were fertilized and frozen for future use. "I feel safe knowing I have those embryos in storage in case I need them," says Margaret.

. . . .

Many chemotherapy drugs are toxic and can damage a woman's egg-producing abilities. Chemotherapy induces cells in the follicles to die, and if a woman loses her follicles, she may go into premature ovarian failure. Younger women have a larger number of follicles and therefore may be able to tolerate the loss of some follicles better than older women. But high doses of chemotherapy or radiation therapy in the pelvic area may cause even a young woman to go into early menopause.

The chemotherapy drug most commonly associated with infertility is cyclophosphamide (Cytoxan). This drug is usually used in combination with other drugs to treat lymphomas, leukemias, and some solid tumors. Combination chemotherapy, which generally uses lower doses of each drug, may be less toxic to the ovaries than chemotherapy with individual drugs. A forty-year-old woman treated with a chemotherapy regimen that includes cyclophosphamide has a 40 percent to 80 percent chance of ovarian failure. Presumably, chemotherapy is less likely to affect follicles when they are not growing. Some studies have suggested that treatment with gonadotropin-releasing hormone (GnRH) agonists during chemotherapy may help young women protect their follicles from being destroyed.

After receiving chemotherapy, a woman can still conceive naturally with no increase in the incidence of birth defects. However, animal studies show an increase in miscarriages and birth defects if pregnancies occur immediately after chemotherapy, probably due to damage to growing follicles. For this reason, we recommend that a woman wait until she is cleared by an oncologist before attempting to become pregnant.

The most common cancer among women of reproductive age is breast cancer. Each year, two hundred thousand women develop breast cancer in the United States, and forty thousand of these are of reproductive age.

Women who have had breast cancer can still safely undergo an IVF procedure. The drug tamoxifen (Nolvadex) both reduces the chances of a recurrence of breast cancer and induces ovulation in a similar manner to clomiphene. One successful IVF protocol for women with breast cancer uses 60 milligrams per day of tamoxifen, starting on cycle day 2 or 3 for five to twelve days. This protocol has more than doubled the yield of embryos compared to nonstimulated IVF, without increasing the risk of cancer recurrence.

Another novel protocol uses letrozole (Femara), a drug that suppresses the conversion of androgens to estrogens. Concomitant use of letrozole and gonadotropins allows for excellent development of several follicles and eggs while keeping estrogen levels low. This is a very good approach for women with estrogen-sensitive tumors, such as breast and uterine cancers.

Conventional IVF ovarian stimulation protocols are usually started at the beginning of a woman's menstrual cycle. If a woman receives a cancer diagnosis at any other time during her cycle, she could wait up to six weeks before it's possible to retrieve her eggs. For many women, six weeks is too long to wait before starting cancer treatment.

Sometimes it may be possible to intervene and program a woman's cycle by using a GnRH antagonist, which may interrupt the woman's own follicle development. Once this is achieved, recombinant FSH can be administered to promote the development of new follicles. The number of eggs obtained using this method is slightly less than those obtained the traditional way, but the egg quality is the same.

Women with early-stage endometrial or ovarian cancers can also preserve their fertility. Stage I endometrial cancer may be treated either with high-dose medroxyprogesterone acetate or megestrol acetate and GnRH analogs. Stage I epithelial ovarian cancer has been treated successfully with fertility-sparing surgery with or without additional chemotherapy.

Radiation Therapy

Women who need pelvic radiation therapy to treat their cancer can protect their ovaries with a procedure called an oophoropexy. In this procedure, a woman's ovaries are surgically positioned outside the proposed radiation field. This is normally done under general anesthesia through an abdominal incision but can also be done under mild sedation through a laparoscope.

A woman's age, the total body area radiated, and the amount of radiation she receives all affect how much her ovaries may be damaged by radiation. A moderate dose of radiation may induce menopause in a woman over forty whereas a younger woman would tolerate a higher radiation dose without going into ovarian failure.

A woman with early-stage cervical cancer can preserve her uterus with a procedure called a trachelectomy. This procedure involves surgically removing the cervix and the lower portion of the uterus that protrudes into the vagina. The rest of the uterus is left in place. The lymph nodes in the pelvis are also removed, usually by laparoscopic surgery, to determine if the cancer has spread. After the cervix is removed, the woman must undergo intrauterine insemination to become pregnant.

Trachelectomy is usually reserved for younger women with early cervical cancer who have small tumors. To prevent immature delivery, a stitch is made at the bottom of the uterus like a drawstring to prevent premature opening of the cervix during pregnancy. After a trachelectomy, a woman has a higher chance of miscarriage, and her baby needs to be delivered by cesarean section. About 70 percent of these women become pregnant.

Ovarian Tissue Freezing

Weill Cornell researchers have been in the forefront of a technique to freeze ovarian tissue and help women preserve their fertility years after ovary-destroying chemotherapy. A Weill Cornell team took a breast cancer patient's ovarian tissue that had been frozen for six years, implanted it under her abdominal skin, and obtained an embryo from eggs collected from the tissue. This unique achievement raised the possibility that women or girls who are about to undergo chemotherapy, radiation, or other ovary-damaging treatments can have their ovaries removed, frozen, and possibly used to restore fertility or reverse menopause at a later date.

Typically, one ovary is removed through a laparoscopic procedure under local anesthesia, and the outer layer of the ovary is cut into strips. These strips are then slowly frozen and preserved in a special solution. The solution dehydrates the ovarian cells and prevents them being damaged by ice crystals forming inside the cells. When the woman wants to become pregnant, the ovarian tissue is thawed rapidly and transplanted under the skin, either in the abdominal area or in the forearm. However, about two-thirds of the eggs will die from a lack of blood flow through the tissue.

Weill Cornell researchers were the first to create an embryo from banked frozen ovarian tissue after ovarian transplantation. Their patient was diagnosed with breast cancer at age thirty and had an ovary removed and frozen. After undergoing chemotherapy that cured her cancer, she had fifteen pieces of ovarian tissue thawed and transplanted under the skin in her abdomen. After three months, the tissue began to produce hormones and eggs, and every month the eggs were collected for an IVF procedure. In eight months, the researchers collected about twenty eggs, and eight of those were good enough to become fertilized. In March 2004, the team reported that they had finally produced an embryo that survived to the healthy, four-cell stage. The embryo was transferred to the patient's uterus, but she didn't get pregnant. At this time, no pregnancies have been reported in humans after subcutaneous tissue transplantation.

Later in 2004, a thirty-two-year-old Belgian woman gave birth to a healthy baby seven years after banking her ovarian tissue before starting chemotherapy for Hodgkin lymphoma. Although she became infertile as a result of the chemotherapy, reimplantation of her ovarian tissue into the pelvic area resulted in ovulation five months later. She became pregnant by natural fertilization eleven months after transplantation of the tissue. There have been seven other pregnancies after pelvic ovarian tissue transplantation after cancer therapy.

These results have opened new perspectives for cancer patients facing premature ovarian failure. Ovarian tissue freezing has become an option for young women diagnosed with cancer. Hundreds of cancer patients around the world have had ovarian tissue frozen in the hope of being able to have children after completing their cancer treatment.

However, freezing ovarian tissue may pose risks. The cancer could return unless the stored ovarian tissue undergoes adequate testing before reimplantation. Fertility centers should have the skills and use the technology needed to check the tissue for residual cancer cells. The concern is that if the ovarian tissue is frozen while the cancer is still active, the tissue could harbor cancer cells. Certain cancers have a high risk of metastases to the ovaries, including leukemias and neuroblastomas, and others pose a moderate risk of metastases, such as advanced breast cancer and adenocarcinoma of the uterus or colon. Other common cancers that hold a low risk of metastases to the ovaries include early-stage breast cancer, Hodgkin lymphoma, non-Hodgkin lymphoma, and squamous-cell carcinoma of the cervix.

When ovarian tissue is thawed, researchers can use several methods to detect residual cancer. They do a histological evaluation to examine the thin strips of tissue and use immunohistochemical staining with antibodies to detect abnormal cells, polymerase chain reaction (PCR), which amplifies sections of DNA, and real-time PCR to detect molecular markers that indicate the presence of cancer cells. Highly sensitive real-time PCR may be the best method of identifying single cancer cells among the hundreds of thousands of normal cells.

As the methods for detecting cancer cells are improving all the time and ovarian tissue can be stored for more than ten years, tests to detect residual disease should be done just before the tissue is transplanted. That means that fertility clinics need to freeze a smaller piece of ovarian tissue separately to be tested later for residual disease.

Ovarian Transplantation

Recently, researchers in St. Louis performed the first successful complete ovary transplantation that led to a live birth. This technique has the potential to preserve fertility for cancer patients who lose ovarian function. Although this technique has also been proposed as a possible way to postpone having children, we strongly feel this technique should be reserved for cancer patients.

The St. Louis team implanted a woman's entire ovary into her thirty-eight-year-old identical twin sister. One of the women had become infertile at the age of fifteen when she suffered premature ovarian failure and went through menopause. Her identical twin, however, remained fertile and agreed to donate an ovary to her sister. Using microsurgical techniques, Dr. Silber attached the ovary to the infertile twin's blood supply and positioned it alongside her fallopian tubes. She began menstruating a few months later and conceived naturally.

Currently, ovarian transplants from one woman to another are generally reserved for identical twins, who share all their DNA. For the operation to work, it is necessary to have a donor who is a precise tissue match. Organs can be transplanted between identical twin sisters without the danger of rejection by the body's immune system and without the immunosuppressant drugs usually necessary to prevent rejection of a transplanted organ. Immunosuppressant drugs can be toxic to the developing fetus and could severely limit the ability to maintain or complete a pregnancy.

Nevertheless, while this technological feat demonstrated superb surgical skill, it should be emphasized that identical twins should be encouraged to undergo egg donation rather than subject themselves to the risks of the major surgery required for ovarian transplantation.

Egg Freezing

Female cancer patients might be good candidates for egg freezing if they have no male partner or have no other fertility options. A frozen-egg procedure may also be indicated for a couple who are struggling with the moral dilemma of what they would do with excess frozen embryos, since no surplus embryos are created.

A growing number of fertility specialists are experimenting with egg freezing as a way to preserve a woman's fertility. But unlike sperm, a woman's eggs are difficult to freeze. It's a tricky process because egg cells have such a high water content, making them susceptible to damage during the freezing and thawing process. A mature egg is also extremely fragile due to its large size and structural complexity.

Harvesting eggs for freezing involves a process similar to that of IVF. For about a month, the woman receives hormone injections to stimulate her ovaries to produce more than one egg. She goes into the fertility clinic every few days for blood tests and ultrasound scans to check her follicles. As with IVF, her eggs are retrieved under sedation with ultrasound guidance and are frozen by the embryologist using a cryoprotectant formula that helps dehydrate the eggs.

Freezing eggs can be performed by traditional slow methods or by a fast freezing method called *vitrification*. The slow freezing method requires a sophisticated machine that sequentially lowers the temperature over time. The faster method uses high concentrations of solutions that allow for an ultrarapid immersion of the egg in liquid nitrogen, creating a glasslike state. Vitrification speeds up the freezing process by six hundred times and prevents the egg from being damaged by ice crystals. The eggs are placed in liquid nitrogen until the woman is ready to use them. Then the eggs are thawed quickly and rehydrated back to their original state.

Only women who are good candidates to go through an IVF procedure should participate in egg freezing. The egg-freezing procedure costs about $15,000, and is not usually covered by health insurance. Annual storage fees run from about $400 to about $1,000.

Egg freezing is not comparable to embryo freezing simply because not all eggs become embryos. Some women are being given false hope that the outcome of egg freezing will be the same as embryo freezing, but there is no guarantee that by freezing your eggs you will someday have a baby. At the moment, your chances are slim. The live-birth rate following fertilization and insemination of frozen eggs is about 4 percent per egg, far less than with frozen embryos. About one thousand babies have been born from frozen eggs worldwide.

Egg freezing was originally introduced as a way of preserving fertility for young single women diagnosed with cancer or other serious conditions that could make them infertile. But it is also marketed as a way to help women delay conception beyond age thirty-five. We and the American Society for Reproductive Medicine Practice Committee believe that egg freezing is still experimental and the procedure should not be offered as a means of deferring reproductive aging. The committee recommends comprehensive counseling for any woman who might be considering egg-freezing services.

The Hope Registry is a patient database that's tracking the safety and efficacy of egg freezing. The registry, sponsored by the drug company EMD Serono, hopes to enroll four hundred women who will go through frozen-egg IVF cycles to identify factors associated with successful frozen-egg outcomes. All of the children born will be monitored for their health and development from birth to first birthday. The study's results should be available in 2013.

Cancer in Men

Many men with cancer at a young age may not have started or completed their family. Cancer treatment can have a number of different effects on men, depending on the duration and dosage of therapy, the treatment regimen, and even the man's age. We often see men who have survived testicular cancer, lymphoma, or leukemia and come to us for fertility treatment. These men are expected to be long-term cancer survivors with a good quality of life.

Men who are infertile appear to have an increased risk of developing testicular cancer. Faulty DNA repair, or errors in the way the body responds to small areas of damage in its genetic material, may contribute to both testicular cancer and infertility. Environmental factors may also play a role in the development of testicular cancer.

Cancer Treatments

Of the 35,000 young men diagnosed with cancer each year, about 90 percent risk losing their fertility to surgery, radiation therapy, or chemotherapy. Surgery for testicular cancer typically includes dissection of lymph nodes around the spine, and this can damage the nerves that control ejaculation. Radiation treatments can affect sperm production. Very low doses of radiation may damage early sperm cells and lead to low sperm counts, although most men recover after a few months. High doses of radiation may cause zero sperm counts (azoospermia).

If a man has only one functioning testicle and cancer is discovered in that testicle, removal of the affected testicle will render the man permanently sterile and require him to take lifelong testosterone treatments to maintain his sex drive and masculinity. Dr. Goldstein has pioneered a microsurgical technique to remove a testicular tumor and preserve the testicle's function. Even if the tumor is too large for the testicle to be preserved, Dr. Goldstein has been able to extract sperm from the normal tissue around the rim of a cancerous testicle that has been surgically removed. These sperm have been frozen and later thawed and used to fertilize eggs with IVF with intracytoplasmic sperm injection (ICSI), resulting in live births.

Many combinations of chemotherapy agents are used to treat cancers commonly found in younger men, including testicular cancer, Hodgkin lymphoma, non-Hodgkin lymphoma, and acute lymphocytic leukemia. The advantage of combination therapy is that doctors can use lower doses of each agent, which reduces the damage to sperm and increases the possibility of restoring sperm production after chemotherapy. Some therapies are more toxic than others. A four-drug combination for Hodgkin lymphoma can lead to azoospermia that lasts for more than ten years, whereas a three-drug combination for testicular cancer may result in long-term azoospermia in less than 20 percent of men.

Even before chemotherapy, a man with cancer may have poor sperm quality. At the time of diagnosis, about three quarters of men with testicular cancer and two thirds of men with Hodgkin lymphoma have below-normal-quality sperm. The tumor in a man's testicle or an undescended testicle, which is often seen in men with testicular cancer, may also lead to abnormal sperm production.

Men who become azoospermic from cancer treatments may still have a chance to father a child. We can usually surgically retrieve sperm from the testicles of 30 percent to 50 percent of the men who had chemotherapy even fifteen or more years ago. Using ICSI, about one third of these men can impregnate their partners, and about 20 percent take home a baby. The success rates are slightly lower than in men with nonobstructive azoospermia due to other reasons.

Several studies show that men who have had cancer therapy have no additional risk for having offspring with congenital abnormalities or birth defects. Other studies suggest that a man may have a higher risk of genetically abnormal sperm within the first year after chemotherapy, so it may be prudent to wait at least one year after completing chemotherapy before trying to have a baby.

Once a cancer survivor has recovered fully, we encourage couples to try to conceive naturally. For those who don't recover their reproductive function, we can offer procedures such as IVF or ICSI.

Sperm Banking

Sperm banking before treatment can help preserve a young male cancer patient's fertility. More than one third of young men with cancer who have banked their sperm succeed in fathering a child using intrauterine insemination (IUI) and half succeed with IVF or ICSI.

When sperm are frozen, the sperm cells enter a state of suspended animation, and all sperm activity is essentially halted until thawing. While the freezing process will kill a significant percentage of sperm, the surviving sperm can be thawed and successfully used for artificial insemination or IVF with ICSI as long as twenty-five years later.

Healthy men who bank sperm usually remain abstinent for two to three days before providing a semen sample. However, cancer patients may not want to delay therapy, so they may collect sperm to be frozen once a day for several days. Also, because they may have poor sperm quality to start with, they may need several samples to produce enough good-quality sperm to bank. In addition, it's unknown whether the banked sperm carries a higher genetic risk, so we recommend genetic counseling for couples to help them understand the potential risks involved.

We recently published our results with 118 couples who underwent 169 cycles of IVF with ICSI with frozen sperm that was banked before the male partner underwent chemo- or radiotherapy. Of the 118 men, 40 percent had testicular cancer, 31.4 percent had lymphoma, 8.5 percent had prostate cancer, and the remaining 20 percent had leukemias, brain cancer, multiple myeloma, bladder cancer, osteosarcoma, and pancreatic or thyroid cancer. Half the patients had abnormal semen parameters after cancer diagnosis and prior to their cancer treatment. There was significant deterioration in their sperm parameters after thawing. Better semen profiles were found in men with lymphomas and other systemic cancers compared to men with testicular and prostate cancers. Semen parameters and success rates were not influenced by how long the sperm were frozen nor the age of the man at cancer diagnosis.

Delivery rates were 50 percent per ICSI cycle, compared to 24 percent when standard IVF was used with thawed sperm prior to the advent of ICSI. In light of the relatively sparse semen available from these men with cancer, we conclude that they should all undergo ICSI. Standard IUI and IVF require much greater—and often unavailable—sperm numbers.

The cost of sperm banking ranges from $200 to $500, plus an additional annual storage fee. Insurance may cover some of these costs.

Sperm Banking by Mail

About 80 percent of young men receive cancer treatments in community hospitals, often in cities that lack sperm banks. Now there is a way for them to bank their sperm by mail. The Live:On kit (http://www.liveonkit.com) is a collaboration between Cryogenic Laboratories, Inc., a sperm-banking facility, Fertile Hope (http://www.fertilehope.org), a nonprofit organization designed to help cancer patients maintain their fertility, and the Lance Armstrong Foundation, the nonprofit group founded by Lance Armstrong and dedicated to empowering cancer patients.

The collection and preservation kit makes it possible for men to send their specimen from anywhere in the continental United States. Each Live:On kit comes complete with the necessary forms, detailed instructions, transport solution, and return shipping information. The transport solution stabilizes the sperm and serves to maintain their quality during transit. Overnight delivery ensures that the sperm bank receives and processes the semen specimen within twenty-four hours.

The kits are available free of charge to oncology health care professionals. Patients pay for the sperm-banking services when they return the kit to the sperm bank. The total cost of the kit is $625. This fee includes $65 for the kit and shipping, $280 for processing, analysis, and freezing, and $280 for storage for one year. Cryogenic Laboratories is donating part of the proceeds from Live:On to Fertile Hope and the Lance Armstrong Foundation. Fertile Hope is offering discounts to financially strapped patients.

The Fertile Hope Web site is also a good resource for both male and female cancer patients to assess their potential for preserving their fertility. A calculator on the site can help both male and female patients and their oncologists determine the risk of infertility according to their cancer type and treatment regimen. Then an options calculator can help plan treatment that protects their future fertility.

More Cancer Doctors Need to Address Fertility

Sperm banking is a simple, accessible, and affordable way for male cancer patients to keep their reproductive options open, yet oncologists do not always offer counseling and education about fertility issues prior to cancer treatment. It may be impossible for doctors to know how important fertility preservation is to cancer patients unless they ask, since patients may not bring up the topic. The cancer diagnosis is such a shock that an issue like fertility is often put on the back burner. Cancer patients tend to be focused on treatment options and survival, and discussions of fertility often are not approached. Surveys show that fewer than 20 percent of young, male cancer patients choose to freeze samples of their sperm before undergoing treatment. Significantly, only a relatively small proportion of men who freeze their sperm ultimately use them to achieve pregnancy.

A national survey of more than six hundred oncologists found that many oncologists do not adequately address fertility issues. The American Society of Clinical Oncology published guidelines in 2006 on how to preserve fertility in cancer patients. The guidelines include discussing a patient's options, referring the patient to fertility specialists, and providing educational materials. Yet the survey results also found that more than one third of the oncologists had no knowledge of the guidelines. Most oncologists say they discuss fertility with their cancer patients, but those talks range widely from a brief mention of risks to an in-depth discussion. In addition, 24 percent of the oncologists say they rarely refer patients to fertility specialists and

60 percent rarely provide educational materials. Oncologists should do more than just talk about preserving fertility; they should provide their patients with the concrete information they need.

In the Future

The holy grail of fertility preservation for women with cancer would be to turn their immature eggs into mature ones. This process is called in vitro maturation (IVM). If this procedure becomes highly successful, we can envision a time when frozen ovarian follicles can be grown and matured in the laboratory without having to transplant a woman's ovary. This would decrease the chance of reintroducing a resident cancer remaining in the frozen tissue of the ovaries and would eliminate the obvious risks involved in surgery. Although IVM from early follicles has been successful in part in animal models, it still has significant hurdles to surmount before it can be applied to humans. Similarly, a boy's testicular tissue may be able to be frozen and matured later in the laboratory to produce sperm.

Eggs Matured from Girls with Cancer

It may be possible to preserve childbearing ability in young girls with cancer. Northwestern University researchers have taken immature ovarian follicles from young female cancer patients and grown them in three-dimensional gels until they became what appear to be good-quality eggs. Their ultimate goal is to be able to freeze the immature follicles, then thaw and mature them in a culture to the point where they are ready to be fertilized.

Similarly, researchers at Hadassah Hebrew University Medical Center in Jerusalem have removed and preserved ovarian tissue from young female cancer patients and then retrieved, matured, and froze eggs from that tissue. They worked with nineteen patients between the ages of five and twenty. On average, they were able to retrieve nine eggs from each patient, and one third of the eggs were successfully matured.

The next step in the Israeli research will be to test the ability of these eggs to become fertilized. None of the eggs has yet been thawed. The real test will come when the girls are ready to have children. The researchers won't know whether the final chapter of this story will have a happy ending until about ten years from now.

Freezing Testicular Tissue in Boys

In boys who have not yet gone through puberty and don't yet produce sperm, testicular tissue can be frozen in the hope that in the future it can be matured in the laboratory to produce sperm. This has been done successfully in mice, but it will likely be a decade or more before this can be accomplished in humans.

Stem Cells

The same stem cell techniques discussed in Chapter 14 can be used to produce sperm or eggs from cancer patients who have no banked tissue or sperm.

Take-Home Messages

- A woman may be able to preserve her fertility by freezing embryos, eggs, or ovarian tissue before she undergoes cancer treatment. Similarly, a man can bank sperm before treatment.
- A woman should wait until she is cleared by an oncologist before trying to conceive.
- Surgical procedures are available to protect a woman's ovaries from exposure to radiation.
- Donor eggs, rather than an ovary transplant, are the more likely fertility treatment if your ovaries are not functioning properly. Egg donation is the only viable option for women who do not freeze embryos, eggs, or ovarian tissue when they develop ovarian failure after cancer treatment.
- Egg freezing is a tricky process and not anywhere near as successful as embryo freezing.
- A man should wait at least one year after completing chemotherapy before trying to impregnate his partner.
- Half of the young men with cancer who bank their sperm are able to father a child through IVF or ICSI.
- If you receive a cancer diagnosis, ask your oncologist how you can preserve your fertility.

Sixteen

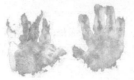

Do Alternative Treatments Work?
Combining Strategies for Fertility Success

. . . .

"Acupuncture is a phenomenal way to relax. When I have the needles in me, I drift off and feel like I'm floating away. I know that the night of my acupuncture treatment I sleep more deeply," says Arnold, a forty-one-year-old television producer. Arnold and his wife, Joan, a forty-year-old reporter, started using acupuncture during their fertility treatments after another couple said the ancient Chinese technique had helped them in their struggle with infertility.

They went to see a woman with a special interest in fertility who had worked with Dr. Goldstein's patients before. "She utilizes acupuncture as well as herbs and lifestyle changes," says Arnold. "She gave me super garlic to help get my blood pressure down a little, Pycnogenol, a bioflavonoid found in tree bark, to improve my sperm count, and linden tea for stress reduction."

Every time Arnold needed to provide a sperm sample for one of the many intrauterine inseminations or in vitro fertilization (IVF) procedures Joan had, he would go for a one-hour acupuncture session. "She had a specific acupuncture protocol to help sperm production," Arnold says. "Other times I'd go to reduce stress or inflammation, or to increase circulation. I had needles in my forehead, my scalp, my ears, my ankles. Each time, she placed the needles in a different place, depending on the treatment for that day."

Joan had six eggs retrieved in her third IVF cycle, and four of them were fer-

tilized with Arnold's sperm. Three embryos were transplanted, and one survived. Their daughter, Jill, is now sixteen months old.

· · · · · · · · · ·

More and more infertile couples are turning to holistic techniques to increase their odds of conception and to cope with the stresses of trying to conceive. There is increasing evidence of the effectiveness of alternative medical approaches. Some fertility clinics, including Weill Cornell, recommend that couples introduce yoga, relaxation, and nutrition into their fertility treatment plans or, in difficult cases, try acupuncture in addition to assisted reproductive technologies (ART).

We recently evaluated the utilization of complementary alternative modalities (CAM) among three hundred of our female patients undergoing infertility treatment. This represents one of the first documentations of the prevalence of CAM usage in infertility patients. The women, average age thirty-seven, had an average duration of infertility ranging from one to five years. The results of anonymous questionnaires showed that they used a range of CAM treatments, primarily acupuncture but also herbal therapy, yoga, massage, special diets, vitamins, stress reduction, and meditation. About half of the women who completed the survey reported using CAM while undergoing ART.

More than 90 percent of the women reported benefits, including stress reduction, improved mood, empowerment, and perceived improved responses, and about three quarters of those who had never used CAM for infertility said they would use it in a future treatment. Despite conflicting reports on the efficacy of CAM, future studies on the effectiveness of these treatments seem warranted.

Traditional Chinese medicine (TCM) believes that both partners should be as healthy as possible at the time of conception to ensure that they have the best possible chance at conceiving. Additionally, TCM aims to improve the overall health of the mother- and father-to-be to decrease the risk of miscarriage. TCM practitioners who work with fertility patients incorporate acupuncture, herbs, and meditative relaxation exercises such as tai chi and qi gong to help balance the body and mind to improve conception rates.

A hectic Western lifestyle may influence fertility through pervasive stress. Studies show that women who participate in mind-body interventions, including yoga, meditation, and visualization, as well as cognitive behavioral therapy, can reduce stress and possibly improve their pregnancy rates. It should be emphasized that it has been difficult to prove that any of these holistic approaches definitely improve your chances of achieving a pregnancy. They are better thought of as adjuncts to fertility treatments.

Traditional Chinese Medicine

TCM practitioners view infertility as a symptom of imbalance, and the goal of therapy is to cultivate balance in body and mind, strengthen the immune system, and create harmony in all areas of life.

One of the principles of TCM is that there are many meridians, or energy pathways through the body, that need to be in balance for good health. Any disruption in these patterns of energy flow, called qi, may lead to disease. For a woman, the goal of therapy is to regulate the menstrual cycle and strengthen her body. TCM practitioners determine which meridians may create problems with fertility or pose a threat to a pregnancy. For a man, the TCM practitioner will ask a series of questions to assess areas that need to be strengthened in order to increase his sperm count and sperm quality.

Like fertility specialists, TCM practitioners first undertake an individual consultation to evaluate a man's or a woman's fertility. Treatment usually lasts for at least three or four months. Be aware that herbal therapy is not recommended during ART cycles.

Various studies have claimed that TCM can be used to regulate the menstrual cycle, regulate hormones by reducing stress, improve blood flow to the ovaries and uterus, improve ovarian function to encourage production of follicles, improve the thickness of the uterine wall lining, reduce uterine contractions after embryo transfer, reduce the chance of miscarriage, and improve sperm parameters and the quality of eggs.

Researchers from Yale University and Chang Gung Institute of Technology in Taiwan reviewed recent studies of TCM in fertility. They found that TCM could regulate gonadotropin-releasing hormone (GnRH) to induce ovulation and improve blood flow to the uterus and improve the menstrual changes of the endometrium. In addition, TCM had an impact on infertility patients with polycystic ovary syndrome, anxiety, stress, and immunological disorders.

However, these were mainly small, uncontrolled studies. The effective dose, side effects, and potential toxicity of TCM in the context of infertility treatment need to be studied in prospective, randomized control trials to demonstrate the safety and effectiveness of TCM treatments.

Acupuncture

Acupuncture involves the insertion of very fine needles into specific points on the body along the meridians to balance the flow of qi.

After reviewing your medical situation and taking a history, an acupuncturist takes your pulse and does an exam to determine your energy state. Then he or she will insert thin, sterile, disposable acupuncture needles into the skin along the meridians at specific positions according to your diagnosis. You lie still for about thirty minutes with the needles in place, as the acupuncturist stimulates the needles manually or with low-voltage electric current or infrared heat. In general, acupuncture treatments for fertility are recommended in courses of once or twice a week for at least three or four months.

Acupuncture is considered a safe procedure, but an inexperienced acupuncturist can potentially cause infection, bleeding, bruising, pain, or even organ puncture when placing the needles. The American Pregnancy Association warns that acupuncture needles inserted into the wrong meridian point may lead to a miscarriage, so you should avoid acupuncture if you are pregnant. The cost of acupuncture ranges from a few hundred to a few thousand dollars, depending on how long you are treated and who is doing the treatment. Many insurance companies cover the cost of acupuncture treatments, but usually not to treat infertility. Check your insurance policy carefully.

As a fertility treatment, acupuncture is said to increase blood flow to the uterus, relax the cervix, and help stabilize the nervous system to allow the body to handle stress better. The effects of acupuncture may also be based on brain chemistry. Acupuncture may help to improve a woman's chances of conceiving by balancing the hormones released by the brain. In 2002, Weill Cornell researchers examined the medical literature and found a clear link between acupuncture treatments and increased production of endorphins, the body's natural painkilling brain chemicals. The studies they reviewed suggested that certain effects of acupuncture are mediated through endorphins, which influence gonadotropin secretion through their action on GnRH and the menstrual cycle. So it's logical to hypothesize that acupuncture may influence ovulation and fertility.

They also found evidence that acupuncture increased blood flow to the uterus and improved the thickness of the uterine lining, which may allow it to be more receptive to implantation. This suggests that acupuncture may provide an excellent alternative for stress reduction in women undergoing infertility treatment.

The Pros and Cons of Acupuncture IVF Studies

The Weill Cornell researchers also noted one prospective, randomized controlled study by researchers at the University of Ulm in Germany that compared the pregnancy rates among 160 women undergoing IVF. Half of the women had acupuncture treatments for twenty-five minutes before and after embryo transfer, and the other half did not. After controlling for confounding variables, the acupuncture group had a significantly higher pregnancy rate (43 percent) than the control group (26 percent).

A more recent review in 2008 led by University of Maryland researchers found that acupuncture might improve the odds of conceiving if done immediately before or after embryo transfer. The analysis pooled results from seven studies on 1,366 women in the United States, Germany, Australia, and Denmark. The women were randomly assigned to receive IVF alone, IVF with acupuncture within a day of embryo transfer, or IVF plus sham acupuncture, in which needles were placed too shallowly or in spots without meridians. One of the studies found acupuncture was beneficial, three studies found a trend in favor of acupuncture, and one study found acupuncture had no benefit. The researchers pooled the results of the smaller studies and found adding acupuncture improved the odds of conception by 65 percent.

But this type of pooled analysis is not proof that acupuncture helps. Since IVF pregnancy rates are at about 50 percent, adding acupuncture might boost a woman's chance of having a baby by about 10 percent. Also, results from these studies should be interpreted with caution. Pregnancy rates without acupuncture varied widely in the different trials and often depended on which country the IVF clinic was in. In clinics where pregnancy rates after IVF were higher, the benefit of acupuncture was smaller. Although this review shows acupuncture has promise, more studies are needed to confirm whether acupuncture can be recommended as an adjunctive treatment alongside IVF.

In contrast, a review in 2009 by researchers at Guy's and St. Thomas' Hospitals in London found that acupuncture may not improve IVF success rates. The researchers analyzed data from fourteen randomized clinical trials involving 2,870 women. Five trials included 877 women who had IVF with or without acupuncture treatments during egg retrieval. Those studies showed no significant difference in the pregnancy rate between those who had acupuncture and those who acted as controls. The other nine trials included 1,993 women who had IVF with or without acupuncture performed at the time of embryo transfer. These studies also reported no substantial difference in pregnancy rates.

Another randomized, prospective study in 2009 by researchers at Boston IVF examined the impact of acupuncture and IVF outcomes. The researchers randomly assigned 150 women about to undergo IVF to have acupuncture or no acupuncture before and after embryo transfer. The women also filled out questionnaires on their anxiety levels and how optimistic they were about the success of the IVF cycle. The acupuncture did not lead to higher pregnancy rates, but those who had acupuncture reported that they were less anxious after the embryo transfer and more optimistic about the outcome of their IVF cycle.

A 2008 Cochrane Collaboration review of data from thirteen studies found no strong evidence that acupuncture improves pregnancy rates, although one study did show a slight increase in the live-birth rate among women who underwent acupuncture on the day of embryo transfer. A number of other recent studies have addressed the use of acupuncture in patients undergoing treatment for infertility. Some show benefit, while others do not.

With all of this conflicting research on acupuncture in IVF, it's hard to know its true effect in improving your chances of taking home a baby. More well-conducted clinical trials are needed to substantiate the use of acupuncture in improving IVF pregnancy rates.

The gold standard of medical testing is the randomized, double-blind clinical trial, in which neither the patients nor the doctors know which treatment is being given. But it may be difficult to do a convincing double-blind trial in a treatment as invasive as acupuncture. The participants have to believe they are being stuck with actual needles. "Placebo" acupuncture with needles that retract into the handle when pressed against the body and don't penetrate the skin might be too realistic and could induce the placebo effect, which means that if you believe that something will work, it really does work. Or the pressure of the placebo acupuncture might induce a response similar to real acupuncture.

That's what researchers at the University of Hong Kong in China found when they looked at real and placebo acupuncture given on the day of embryo transfer in 370 patients in a randomized, double-blind trial. A trained acupuncturist applied the placebo acupuncture to the same acupuncture points as in the real acupuncture. Surprisingly, the researchers found that the overall pregnancy rate for the placebo acupuncture was significantly higher (55 percent) than for the real acupuncture (44 percent).

They speculate that the placebo acupuncture acted like acupressure, a form of acupuncture that uses manual pressure on the meridian points instead of needles pushed into the points. Blood tests showed that women in both groups had a decrease in the stress hormone cortisol and lower levels of anxiety. That may have increased their chances of conception. The researchers admit they cannot draw firm conclusions about the study because they did not compare the two groups with a third, control group of patients who did not receive either form of acupuncture.

The bottom line is that the jury is still out as to whether acupuncture can help increase your chances of getting pregnant with IVF. There are still some unresolved issues, but it's unlikely that acupuncture does any harm, and it probably does reduce the stress associated with fertility treatment. If you do decide to try acupuncture, always check on the training and qualifications of the acupuncturist. The National Certification Commission for Acupuncture and Oriental Medicine (http://www.nccaom.org/find/index.html) can help you locate a board certified, licensed acupuncturist in your area.

Chinese Herbs

Many Chinese herbal therapies are said to improve the chances of conception. The herbs address underlying imbalances so that the body can function more healthfully. In the treatment of infertility, herbs are used to promote hormone balance, improve sperm and egg quality, regulate the menstrual cycle, enhance mucus secretions, tone the uterus, nourish the endometrial lining, and maintain pregnancy.

TCM herbal therapy generally uses combinations of herbs. Each herbal prescription is uniquely tailored to a patient's detailed health history. The formula is carefully balanced to accentuate the patient's strengths and to reduce the possibility of side effects. The different herbs combined in a formula can be made into teas (decoctions), powders, or pills.

Chinese herbs offered to women for the treatment of infertility include damiana, dong quai, chaste tree, ginseng, and hachimijiogan. Chinese herbs used to treat male infertility include deer antler, rehmannia, gui-zhi-fu-ling-wan, bushen shengjing pill, ju jing powder, hachimijiogan, and ninjinotoh.

TCM herbalists have extensive training and clinical experience and do not encourage self-medication, which may be harmful or even fatal. They claim to be able to treat infertility effectively and believe that herbs cause fewer side effects than fertility drugs, but they usually are willing to work in conjunction with conventional medical treatments.

The mechanisms of how Chinese herbal therapy works is not well understood. One possibility is the herbs act as antioxidants as well as anti-estrogens. Researchers at the University of Kent in England studied the biochemical activity of Chinese herbs commonly used in the treatment of male infertility, including thirty-seven individual herbs and seven herb decoctions. They found a range of strong to weak antioxidant and antiestrogen effects. Since the process of sperm formation is under strict hormonal control, and oxidative stress, which causes the formation of free radicals, has been implicated in male infertility, this is a plausible mechanism of action for Chinese herbs.

Other Herbal Therapies

Herbal therapies have been part of folk medicine throughout history. They can be made from roots, leaves, bark, fruits, and flowers, and are most effective when they are fresh. In the United States, plants are classified as foods or food additives and are not regulated by the Food and Drug Administration. They can be found in abundance in health food stores and grocery stores.

Herbs are used to improve fertility and provide nutrients for the uterus, regulate hormones, improve the regularity of the menstrual cycle, improve sperm quality and health, and increase libido. Among the more common herbs used to help regulate menstrual cycles and ovulation and treat female infertility are black cohosh, vitex agnus-castus, false unicorn root, red clover blossom, licorice, wild yam, sarsaparilla, and thistle. Common herbs prescribed to men to boost fertility and regulate male hormones include saw palmetto, Panax ginseng and American ginseng, astragalus, sarsaparilla, and yohimbe. A pine tree bark extract, sold under the brand name Pycnogenol, which is rich in antioxidants, has been shown to improve the sperm quality and function in a small study of nineteen men who took the extract for ninety days.

Your best bet is probably to seek out the advice of a qualified herbal practitioner. A properly trained herbalist or naturopath can best recommend a formula of herbs to address your health history and fertility problems and provide you with high-quality herbs.

It is important that you tell your fertility specialist that you are using herbal therapy. Many herbs have active ingredients that can cause adverse effects when mixed with prescription or over-the-counter drugs. Certain herbs can interfere with anesthesia or lead to complications. Some herbs should not be taken during pregnancy because they may be harmful to your growing fetus. It is important that you understand the benefits and risks of herbal therapy before using any natural therapies to address your infertility.

Claims for the benefits of herbal remedies are based mostly on anecdotes or observational studies. Well-designed, randomized, controlled trials to evaluate the efficacy, mechanism of action, and toxicities of herbal therapies are needed to substantiate these approaches as fertility treatments. *In general, we do not prescribe herbal therapy.*

Stress and Conception

A body of evidence continues to build about the effects of chronic stress on a woman's ovulation and a man's sperm production. Chronic stress alters brain signals to the hypothalamus, which in turn affects the hypothalamus's signals to the pituitary and the pituitary's signals to the ovaries and testicles. Stress may lead to a cascade of hormonal events that lead to inhibition of the body's central reproductive hormone signal, GnRH, and subsequently disturb ovulatory function or sperm production and sexual activity.

Chronic stress, whether emotional or physical, taxes the body and has been linked to infertility. Humans are designed to endure acute stress. That's a part of life. But the significant amount of stress couples endure, cycle after cycle, as they attempt to conceive may disrupt reproductive function. Normal fitness and diet routines may fall by the wayside, leading to a more frazzled, stressed lifestyle. Putting this into Eastern philosophic terms, if you are not in harmony with yourself and your culture, you are stressed.

Stressful life events have been associated with poor IVF outcome. The majority of infertility research focuses on stress related to IVF. It's still unclear whether naturally occurring stress influences IVF pregnancy chances. In their study of 809 women undergoing IVF, researchers at the University of Aarhus in Denmark found that women were more likely to become pregnant if they had less stress in their lives in the month before they came in for IVF. Not surprisingly, they noted high amounts of stress around the time of egg retrieval.

Other research shows that many women suffer anxiety and depression after a failed IVF attempt, which also isn't surprising. However, in studies attempting to make a direct connection between stress and lower IVF success rates, the results are mixed. We still need more information to determine the exact relationship between stress and its effect on IVF success. It may be helpful for you to know that anxiety or depression won't necessarily ruin your chances of having a baby.

Stress and Sperm

Sperm production takes two and a half to three months from the time sperm-cell precursors start to divide until mature sperm enter the semen at the time of ejaculation. Randomized controlled studies in animals have clearly shown that chronic, unremitting stress will render male rats sterile and reduce testosterone production as well.

Although human studies cannot be as strictly randomized and controlled for ethical reasons, the research that has been done strongly suggests that stress can decrease sperm production and impair sperm quality. Because sperm production takes so long, stressful events may result in impaired sperm counts and quality up to three months later.

The same mind-body techniques that may enhance female fertility might also enhance male fertility. In addition, a reduction in stress is also likely to reduce use of gonadotoxins such as alcohol, cigarettes, and recreational drugs. Stress reduction techniques such as regular exercise, meditation, or a calming environment are likely to enhance male fertility as well as general health.

Mind-Body Therapy

If you feel you are under stress, a mind-body approach may help you to cope better. A mind-body approach is based on the premise that each person should be treated as a whole and that the mind and body are integrated. What affects the body affects the mind, and what affects the mind affects the body.

Many alternative medicine practitioners hold to the belief that a mind-body approach can help men and women reclaim their bodies as their own, diminish stress, and increase a sense of well-being. All mind-body approaches focus on strengthening and integrating the connections between the emotional and the physical to reestablish a sense of control, help resolve loss, and assist in moving on with life. Addressing the emotional and psychological issues that often accompany infertility can also help couples feel that they are taking an active role in regaining positive feelings about themselves and their lives.

Mind-body approaches can complement medical treatments for infertility and can strengthen your resolve as you embark on the next medical procedure with renewed energy. Relaxation techniques, including meditation, yoga, mindfulness training, spiritual exploration, and journal writing, are all methods used by alternative medicine to help infertile couples achieve peace of mind. One technique may work better for you than another, so it may be worth trying out a few.

Many people use alternative therapies to resolve fertility problems, but it's not clear whether they use them to reduce stress or to increase their chances of getting pregnant. So researchers from the University of Wales in the United Kingdom and the University of Copenhagen in Denmark set out to study why women made the choice to use these therapies. They examined the psychosocial and medical profiles of 818 Danish women at the start of IVF treatment and then looked at which women went on to use alternative therapies over the subsequent year. Women who went on to use alternative therapies such as reflexology and nutritional supplements during their treatments were more distressed and emotionally affected by their fertility problems than those who did not use alternative therapies.

This may mean that the women who were using alternative therapies had greater stress even before treatment.

It makes sense to try to relieve the stress of infertility, but there may be better ways to do this than through the use of alternative therapies. For example, some infertile couples who have gone through a relatively simple, inexpensive, sixteen-week program of cognitive behavioral therapy have found they could have a baby with little need for infertility drugs and procedures. This type of brief coping strategy may be more appealing if you don't want to use conventional one-on-one or group counseling to reduce stress.

Yoga and Exercise

More women, and some men, are turning to yoga to complement traditional Western medical treatments for fertility. A moderate exercise program can help you achieve and maintain a fertile body weight, decrease stress, promote good hormonal regulation, and increase self-esteem. Yoga is certainly a fertility-friendly exercise, and yoga classes designed to promote fertility are said to increase blood flow to the reproductive organs, regulate hormone function, and lower stress.

The idea behind yoga is the simple movement of energy using poses to correct blockages or imbalances in the body. Certain yoga poses designed to enhance fertility include the bridge pose, the child's pose, the cobbler's pose, and the legs on the wall pose. Yoga poses work by stretching muscles and realigning the body. They purportedly benefit fertility by stretching and opening tight pelvic muscles to increase blood flow to the ovaries and uterus.

In addition to the physical stimulation, much of yoga's beneficial effect on fertility comes from the deep, mindful breathing that is an integral part of any yoga practice. Yoga breathing is an effective way to relax and may decrease levels of the stress hormone cortisol. If a few yoga classes don't relax you, then move on to a different form of relaxation therapy. You'll find more relaxation techniques in Chapter 17.

Yoga may give you back the sense that your body can make you feel good. Practicing yoga with your partner may also help strengthen the bond between the two of you and bring you closer together.

In the Future

Lasers have become an important tool for infertility surgeons, allowing them to focus a greater amount of energy in a smaller area than ordinary light. Now some acupuncturists are using low-energy laser beams instead of traditional acupuncture needles to direct the flow of energy at acupuncture points. A laser acupuncturist typically aims a beam of light from a laser tube onto an acupuncture point, stimulating it in a similar way to acupuncture needles.

Presented at a national meeting, the first large clinical trial of laser acupuncture shows significantly higher implantation rates, but only slightly highly pregnancy rates, when women had laser acupuncture treatments before and after embryo transfer during IVF. A New Jersey Medical School researcher led a study that divided one thousand women into five groups. The first group received traditional acupuncture. The second group received laser acupuncture with a red-beam laser with shallow penetration. The third group had placebo laser acupuncture. The fourth group relaxed in a dimly lit room with soft music. The last group received no treatment.

All of the treated patients received one treatment at traditional acupuncture points for twenty-five minutes before and after embryo transfer. The study was double-blinded in a way: the laser was preprogrammed either to fire for the treatment group or not to fire for the placebo group, and the acupuncturist could not tell if the laser had fired.

The implantation rate was 34 percent in the laser acupuncture group compared to 25 percent to 30 percent in the other groups. Clinical pregnancy rates were higher with laser acupuncture at 55 percent, but not much more than the 44 percent to 52 percent for the other groups, including 50 percent in the group who received no treatment.

The researchers feel that laser acupuncture could help improve outcomes during IVF, but they believe that a great deal more study is needed to determine the best protocol for acupuncture therapy, laser or otherwise, in patients undergoing infertility treatments.

Take-Home Messages

- The goal of traditional Chinese medicine is to balance your body and mind, strengthen your immune system, and harmonize your life.
- Acupuncture treatments for fertility are usually once or twice a week for at least three or four months.
- Studies show both positive and negative results on whether acupuncture can increase your chances of getting pregnant with IVF.
- Chinese herbalists personalize therapy for your particular form of infertility. Using these herbs on your own may be harmful. We usually do not recommend this form of treatment.
- If you consult an herbal therapist, make sure your fertility specialist knows what herbs you are using. We do not generally prescribe herbal therapy.
- Studies on whether stress affects your ability to conceive with IVF are inconclusive.
- Stressful events may impair your sperm count and quality for up to three months.
- Relaxation techniques such as meditation, yoga, mindfulness training, spiritual exploration, and journal writing may help you reduce stress.

Seventeen

What About the Rest of My Life?

The Emotional Side of Fertility Issues

. . . .

"The emotions of a fertility cycle are like a rocket launch—they could go in a dif-ferent direction in an instant," says Michael, a forty-seven-year-old businessman. "Every part of the process is emotionally draining. For guys, the biggest issue is producing sperm samples. When I was twenty, I could have done it while I was being shot at. It's a lot harder when you're in your forties and everything is riding on the outcome, particularly on the day of in vitro fertilization (IVF). And we feel terribly judged, particularly if the sample is only so-so."

Michael spoke to a Weill Cornell psychologist to help him feel more comfort-able producing a sperm sample for an IVF cycle. "She suggested I think of ways to become more comfortable with the process and also gave me a relaxation tape," he says. "I prepacked a water bottle, a headset and my iPod, and brought them with me the day we were scheduled for IVF. The routine made me comfortable and helped me relax."

. . . .

The inability to reproduce touches the very essence of a couple as a man and a woman, husband and wife, sexual partners, and members of society. Some consider becoming parents as a right of passage into adulthood. The impressive number of medical technologies now available to diagnose and treat infertility offer great hope to infertile couples. At the same time, years of failed medical therapies and disappointing outcomes can take a tremendous emotional toll on couples who must go to extraordinary lengths to bear a child. Infertility becomes a life crisis.

The need to conceive a child is compelling, so it's not surprising that many couples will go to any length to fulfill their dreams of having a baby. When a couple is unable to have a child, they may experience a range of feelings, including depression, anxiety, anger, isolation, guilt, and helplessness. Infertility can result in lowered self-esteem, undermine marital and sexual relations, and place a strain on relationships with family and friends, as well as cause significant financial hardships.

The evaluation and treatment of infertility may themselves be difficult for some couples to handle emotionally. As couples go through IVF, they become acutely aware that this may be their last chance for pregnancy. The egg retrieval can be particularly stressful on a woman anxious to produce enough viable eggs, and the semen collection may put emotional pressure on the man to perform and provide a good-quality sperm sample. Embryo transfer is usually a very emotional time because at that point the outcome is out of the couples' control. The two-week wait for the pregnancy test at the end of an IVF cycle is often fraught with emotional tension.

With the rapid growth of assisted reproductive technologies (ART), infertile couples have more treatment opportunities for creating a family. These opportunities, however, can bring additional stresses as couples grapple with difficult decisions about last-chance treatments, including donor egg or sperm or opting for adoption. The seemingly endless treatment options make it even more difficult for couples to know when to end treatment.

Emotional Responses to Infertility

Many couples experience infertility with the same grief associated with the death of a loved one. In fact, infertile couples may be just as depressed and anxious as patients who have cancer, heart disease, or AIDS. The whirlwind of emotions that infertility brings can feel overwhelming. Knowing that your feelings are normal may help you better understand them.

Depression

Infertile men and women often say they feel sad or tired. They can't eat or sleep, they're anxious, irritable, or pessimistic. These are all symptoms of depression. Women often have a short bout of depression around a specific event—they get their period (again), attend a baby shower or holiday party, or find out a friend is pregnant. This is a normal response to the emotional pain of infertility. However, if the depression becomes severe, and you begin to feel hopeless, can't perform daily functions, and have suicidal thoughts, seek help from a mental health professional.

Guilt

Many women feel they are the cause of the couple's infertility, although their male partners may be responsible for the problem in at least half of the cases. They feel personally responsible for their infertility, and become obsessed with searching their past for the potential cause—was their job too stressful or did they postpone pregnancy too long to foster their careers. Men with male-factor infertility may also feel guilty, but they are often reluctant to share their disappointment and grief because they feel it will only add to the stress of the situation. A man may feel particularly guilty for not being able to carry on his family's name.

Isolation

Our society places a high premium on having a family. A couple may begin to feel isolated when they realize they are unable to do what other couples do so easily and naturally. Each month of "trying" without getting pregnant feels like a personal failure. People who haven't experienced infertility may not understand the emotional pain and may make insensitive or rude remarks. Some couples decide to insulate themselves from the pain brought on by birthday parties or family gatherings or even avoid any activities that involve children. These feelings of isolation can significantly lower your self-esteem.

Anger

Some couples become angry. Life is so unfair! This anger often stems from feeling powerless and usually masks anxiety, fear, and anguish. Most infertile couples have grown up with the notion that if they work hard enough and are "good," they will be rewarded. But there is no foolproof recipe for success with infertility. You may feel hurt and frustrated that you can't control this part of your lives.

Infertility and Stress

For many couples, infertility becomes a part of every waking moment. It dictates decisions regarding jobs, vacations, and family get-togethers. Many patients describe themselves as feeling "stuck" or as if their lives are out of control. Others feel they are on an emotional roller coaster. The ride shifts from hope one day to despair the next. The intense feelings may overpower you as you strive to cope with the ups and downs of the infertility journey.

Studies suggest that stress, depression, and anxiety may affect a woman's odds of having a successful pregnancy. So it's important to understand how to ease stress as you undergo fertility treatment. The healthier you are, the better able your brain will be to cope with stress. The more you know about your condition, its causes, and treatments, the less stress you will feel about it.

Stress may not directly cause infertility, but the two are definitely related. High levels of stress may affect a woman's levels of estrogen and progesterone and may also cause irregular ovulation. Chronic stress may develop with the continuing cycle of hopefulness at the beginning of each menstrual period followed by despair with each new period. Research shows that depressed women may have lower pregnancy rates than nondepressed women.

And men may also be affected. Other research shows men with previously normal sperm counts are more likely to have low sperm counts after a year or more of infertility. Men may also face the stressful situation where they have to produce a sperm sample on demand. Freezing one or two semen samples as a backup prior to an IVF retrieval can help eliminate this fear of failure. The knowledge that there are sperm frozen as an emergency backup usually guarantees it will never have to be used.

Coping with Stress

The Weill Cornell psychological services team runs a two-hour evening stress-management group to help couples undergoing ART procedures. Group members learn relaxation techniques, assertiveness skills, and other helpful ways to manage emotional distress.

You, too, can learn coping strategies to help you manage the stress of infertility and restore a sense of control to your lives. Mind-body approaches, if practiced regularly, can help you manage the effects of stress. The following stress-management techniques can be tools to reduce anxiety and regain a feeling of hope about your fertility treatments.

Breathing Exercises. Practice breathing in slowly through your nose for a count of six, then breathing out slowly for a count of eight. As you slow your breaths, your mind will become quiet and your body will relax. Focused breathing can help you reduce anxiety and tension.

Journal Writing. Write in a personal journal for ten minutes each day. Putting your thoughts and feelings down on paper provides an emotional catharsis, helps you gain insight, and can improve your physical and mental health.

Meditation and Relaxation. Focus your mind on one thought, phrase, or prayer for twenty minutes at a time. This repetition can lead to the "relaxation response," a state of complete relaxation that can help balance mental and physical health.

Mindfulness. Practice living in the moment. This form of "mindfulness" allows you to focus fully and engage yourself in only one activity at a time. Mindfulness can give you a greater appreciation of everything in life.

Make Time for Yourself. Make time to enjoy yourself at least once a day. Make a list of twenty things that bring you pleasure, whether it's taking a walk, treating yourself to dinner at your favorite restaurant, listening to your favorite music, getting a massage, lighting a scented candle, taking an afternoon nap, or reading a book on something besides infertility. Taking a break to carve out some personal time can help to recharge your emotional and physical energy.

Managing Negative Thoughts

Stress is often caused by negative thoughts, and these thoughts create moods that can lead to physical reactions and behaviors. You can learn to identify negative thoughts and replace them with more balanced thoughts or affirmations. Individuals and couples can learn cognitive restructuring, which is the basis of cognitive behavior therapy and provides a way for dealing with negative, self-defeating thoughts and irrational beliefs. Cognitive restructuring interrupts this negative cycle to help you identify your negative thoughts, question how valid they are, and then replace them with new, more balanced thoughts.

Here are some examples from our psychological services team.

The next time you think . . .	Stop and replace it with . . .
"I waited too long."	"I wasn't ready before. Now my husband and I are in a better position both financially and emotionally."
"I'll never have a baby."	"I can't predict the future. I haven't had success yet, but my doctors are optimistic and I am doing everything that I can to pursue treatment and become a mother."
"I can't do anything right, even get pregnant."	"I've had many successes in my life. I'm doing everything I can to optimize my chances, but some things are out of my control."
"I'll never be happy or feel complete without a child."	"I must remember that I was many things before this life crisis. I am not merely an 'infertile woman' but a woman who is struggling with infertility. If infertility treatment doesn't work, it doesn't mean I can't have a child. There are other ways to build a family such as egg donation and adoption."

Two other ways to reduce stress are yoga and acupuncture. These ancient arts may help you reduce stress during fertility treatments, and possibly improve your fertility as well (see Chapter 16). And regular aerobic exercise is a great stress reducer for both men and women. To help reduce stress, exercise for twenty to forty minutes three to four times a week at an intensity that makes you sweat.

How Men and Women Respond to Infertility

Men and women tend to respond quite differently to infertility. In general, women tend to express their emotions, while many men unconsciously suppress their feelings in an effort to console and comfort their partners. Some women become obsessed with talking about having a baby; men tend to cope by using denial, distancing, avoidance, and withdrawal. Typically, the woman wants her husband to be more emotional, and the man wants his wife to be more rational.

Studies show that women tend to experience greater levels of distress than their male partners in terms of anxiety, depression, and hostility as well as more stress and lower self-esteem. Often it's the woman who has to bear the brunt of the medical interventions. She has to show up for regular monitoring and go through the day-to-day struggle of hormone injections, drug side effects, and recurring periods. Women, more than men, tend to express higher levels of depression about infertility. Infertile women tend to feel more distress than infertile men, and women report that they feel more stress than men during IVF treatment.

Little information exists on the association between infertility and depression or reduced quality of life in men. When Weill Cornell doctors examined thirty-nine men of an average age of thirty-eight who came in for an infertility evaluation, they found that most of the men reported a significantly lower quality of life, and almost one third had documented depression. Not surprisingly, the younger the man, the more likely he was to be depressed about his infertility.

There is a common belief that being unable to father a child is shameful and emasculating. Men with male-factor infertility tend to have anxiety and loss of self-esteem. And infertile men may suffer distress just as much as women, according to British researchers. Researchers at Cardiff University in Wales measured the psychological health of more than 250 couples with male-factor infertility, female-factor infertility, mixed causes, or unexplained infertility; couples were assessed before the start of treatment and one year later. The men felt mental and physical stress, had marital distress, and struggled to cope with infertility over time, and men in all four groups suffered equally.

Sex and Infertility

When a couple can't conceive, sexual intercourse may become mechanical and thought of as "sex on demand." Couples feel they are obligated to be sexually active on the optimal fertile days of a woman's cycle. Many infertile couples say they suffer from a lack of desire or get little sexual pleasure. Some begin to associate sex with failure and avoid it whenever possible.

Making love is one of the best ways for a couple to connect emotionally, but not if their sex lives are associated with frustration, anger, and resentment. If you and your partner are experiencing sexual dissatisfaction, you might consider consulting a professional counselor to help you regain a more positive, enjoyable sex life during fertility treatments. If you have any sexual dysfunction, then a consultation with a sex therapist may be appropriate.

Infertility can actually strengthen your marriage and bring you closer to your partner. Often, you must cope together and support each other. In fact, few couples divorce because of infertility.

As you face the relentless struggle to have a baby, it's crucial to keep lines of communication open during difficult times. Effective communication is important during stressful situations. It's also important to learn how to communicate assertively and to understand nonverbal communication, such as body language, eye contact, and actions. University of Copenhagen researchers studied 2,250 infertile men and women at the beginning of infertility treatment and one year later. The men who actively confronted their infertility by letting their feelings out and asking others for advice continued to have good marital relationships.

Coping with Family and Friends

Infertility may cause a tremendous amount of strain on relationships with family and friends. Some families and friends are supportive, while others just add to your stress. This may make you angry or cause you to isolate yourselves from them. You may feel jealous of friends and relatives who have babies. Friends and relatives may aggravate the situation by repeatedly asking you when you plan to have a baby, or by unwittingly talking endlessly about their own children. Family gatherings may be particularly painful as you deal with loss and grief.

The constant questioning and advice offered by family and friends can increase your stress level. They may ask you about the details and costs of procedures or minimize your situation by saying "Just relax" or "Take a vacation." Or they may blame your infertility on your career and suggest you quit your job or work fewer hours to limit your stress.

Some family members may want to help but don't know what to do or say, while others may prefer to avoid the topic completely. Many people feel uncomfortable discussing infertility because it relates to having sex. The older generation may be ignorant of modern technology and new methods of conception. Siblings and friends may flaunt their own fertility, intentionally or unintentionally.

If you feel a lack of understanding, you may not want to go home for the holidays or may decide to avoid anything having to do with children. But you shouldn't sacrifice your social networks just when you need them the most. If you put a temporary limit on contact with insensitive family members and friends, seek out help from other, more supportive friends and family members, therapists, or online or in-person infertility support groups.

Most couples struggle with what details of treatment to reveal. A family gathering may be the right time to share your experiences with family members. You might speak to one or two family members ahead of time and let them spread the word or you may decide simply to answer probing questions honestly. Be aware of who is capable of being understanding and supportive, and increase your time with those people. Reduce your time with those who cannot provide the support you need. You may be surprised to find that the family members and friends you have always relied on for comfort may not be the same people that you turn to during this particular life crisis.

Family, friends, and even strangers may ask insensitive questions. If you have anticipated a question and rehearsed a response, you are more likely to be able to answer quickly and change the subject. Come up with one or two standard answers that make it clear that you do not wish to discuss the topic. For example, when someone asks, "When are you going to have children?" your response may be, "We're working on it!"

In some cases, friends and family members just need to be educated about infertility and how it's treated. They may also need to know how they can support you. Tell them what is helpful and what is harmful. For example, you may ask them not to invite you to socialize with friends or family members who are pregnant or who have new babies. Specifying what you want from them can give you a sense of control.

Many family members and friends struggle with how to support a couple experiencing infertility. They may feel entitled to touch on private, painful areas with intrusive questions and well-intended advice. Tell them their support and interest are appreciated, but not their advice on how to get pregnant. You've educated yourselves about infertility and are capable of making your own decisions about your fertility treatment.

Use communication and empathy to your benefit. Express yourself—with humor if possible—and don't lock your feelings inside. Share your feelings about family and friends and how they are affecting you with your partner. Together you can make it through. Try to understand your partner's feelings. You don't have to agree with your partner, but see if you can put yourself in his or her shoes. Then see if you can find ways to compromise so that both of you can fulfill your emotional needs.

Secondary Infertility

· · · · · · · · · ·

After her son, Andrew, was born with Dr. Goldstein's help, Liz, a thirty-six-year-old entrepreneur, waited two years before trying to get pregnant again with her husband, Carl, a thirty-eight-year-old schoolteacher. She did become pregnant—three more times—but each time ended in a miscarriage. "By the time I was approaching forty, Carl and I decided against IVF. I couldn't take that much time away from my business," says Liz. Instead they looked into adoption, and a year later brought Carla into their family. "It's been ten years since we adopted our darling Carla," says Liz. "But I still look back and wonder whether we should have tried harder to have another baby."

· · · · · · · · · ·

Secondary infertility, the inability to conceive or carry a pregnancy after one or more successful pregnancies, can be a baffling, difficult emotional experience. Like couples with primary infertility, couples with secondary infertility have similar feelings of guilt, denial, depression, and anxiety. And they have the added stress of worrying about the effect the infertility experience is having on their existing child or children.

Couples with secondary infertility are in the unique position of being both biologic parents and infertile. They often describe themselves as experiencing the joys of parenthood while at the same time feeling deprived because they can't have another child. They may feel grateful for the child or children they have but also yearn for another. These couples may delay seeking medical treatment if previous pregnancies came easily. They assume it will eventually happen again. But as a woman ages, she has less and less chance of conceiving. When a woman doesn't get pregnant, she may chide herself for not having sought treatment sooner.

Some patients with secondary infertility feel resentful of those who have a second or a third child and also feel guilty because they are unable to provide their child with a sibling. They tend to feel different from families with several children. But a family of three is still a "normal" family.

Couples with secondary infertility often feel social pressure to have more than one child, yet they may also be told by friends and family that they should "just be thankful for what they have." This internal conflict can lead to lingering ambivalent feelings and a rehashing of what could have been.

As with primary infertility, couples with secondary infertility may benefit from individual or couples' counseling or from participating in patient support groups aimed at assisting couples who are experiencing secondary infertility.

Support Groups

"When I couldn't get pregnant after my third attempt at IVF, I felt like my life was spinning out of control," says Nancy, a forty-year-old doctor. "It was driving me crazy. I admit I'm high strung and used to getting what I want. But no matter how hard I tried, I wasn't able to get the results I wanted."

Nancy and her husband Walter sought out help from a psychologist at Weill Cornell. "The psychologist showed me how to let go of what I couldn't control. Now I do breathing exercises or listen to a visualization tape every day. She gave us a plan. I'm doing better, and feel more in control," says Nancy.

. . . .

In our practice at Weill Cornell, we offer two types of support groups for our couples. The drop-in group is a confidential group in an informal atmosphere where you can obtain information and support while coping with the stresses of infertility. Some women come in while waiting for their daily blood work or ultrasound appointment. The first half of the group is led by our psychologists, and the second half of the group is led by our nursing team leader.

The group is offered once a week for one hour in the IVF suite. A lot of out-of-town patients tend to join the drop-in group, which usually has up to ten people each session. Only about 20 percent of our patients reach out for psychological services, although more could probably benefit from them. Couples are often more willing to ask for help after their second or third IVF cycle as they begin to become more depressed and anxious.

The second group is a stress-management group that is open to couples interested in learning lifestyle and behavioral skills to help identify and manage emotional stress. The psychologist meets with up to fifteen people for two hours once a week for six to eight weeks. The couples learn about the connection between the mind and the body, cognitive restructuring skills, and how to elicit the relaxation response. The things they are used to relying on to reduce stress—caffeinated beverages, exercise, deep massage, long baths—are stripped away and replaced with other tools, including visualization and progressive muscle relaxation. These skills give our couples a renewed sense of hope and control over the often out-of-control experience of dealing with infertility.

Even if you can't get to Weill Cornell, a wide variety of psychotherapeutic treatment approaches can be highly effective in helping infertile patients cope. You and your partner may consider going to a therapist for brief focused therapy, behavioral therapy (including stress management), crisis intervention, or grief counseling.

For many couples, if they have never been in counseling before, infertility could be the one reason that brings them to see a professional counselor.

Infertility can strain a marriage, rip apart communications between partners, and challenge their sense of identity. Some couples need extra help to get through it. Even those who have been in analysis for many years may feel their regular therapist doesn't quite understand the feelings that underlie infertility, so they come in for additional work with our fertility counselors.

In an ideal world, every couple we see would have at least one session with one of our three psychologists to learn what to expect emotionally from their fertility treatment. This type of "implications counseling" is mandated in Canada. In the United States, the only couples who *must* meet with a counselor are those considering third-party pregnancy with egg donation, embryo donation, sperm donation, or a surrogate pregnancy.

We encourage our couples to focus on the relationship with their partners and to try to communicate with each other in a mutually supportive way. We also give them the chance to speak to other couples with the same fertility issues who have already gone through the treatments. And we suggest they try our in-house support groups, as well as patient advocacy support groups or online support groups.

As we have seen in our drop-in group, psychosocial counseling may be more readily accepted after repeated treatment failure and in the later stages of treatment when a couple's social networks may have begun to weaken. We have found that in particular men who come in for counseling show an improvement in their mental well-being and their perception of what it means to be infertile.

End-of-Treatment Strategies

With fertility treatment options now seemingly endless, the decision on when to end treatment becomes increasingly difficult. You and your partner may find it helpful to set limits on how many and what kinds of procedures you can handle or afford. Discuss with your partner what options you might consider, such as third-party pregnancy, adoption, or accepting that you will have no children. Deciding on a plan will help reduce your anxiety during fertility treatments and ameliorate feelings of hopelessness. Know where you can find support groups or a fertility counselor to help you grieve if fertility treatments do fail.

Keep a record of the costs of your fertility treatments, which can mount up with each attempt to achieve a pregnancy because most procedures are not covered by insurance companies. This will help prevent repeated fertility treatments draining you both financially and emotionally.

Unfortunately, not all infertile couples who go through ART treatments take home a baby. At that point, it's important for you to redefine success. Your fertility specialist and psychological counselor can help you make the decision to end treatment and help you reformulate your personal definition of success. As health care professionals in the fertility field, we are deeply invested in assisting a couple to have a healthy baby. We also feel personal disappointment and a sense of loss when that doesn't happen. Fortunately, as medical technology continues to improve, we are able to reframe what success means.

If you are considering third-party reproduction, then you must both agree that this is your best alternative to becoming parents. When you make the conscious decision to stop fertility treatment, you redefine what "family" means to you. You must address the emotional consequences of not conceiving a child and must grieve for the genetically shared child you had hoped for. This difficult, emotionally charged process may raise intense feelings of loss that you must both work through.

It's likely that you've been thrust into an intense crisis at various points in your infertility experience, such as a failed ART cycle or bad news about your future treatment options. The emotional stress of failing to conceive can be devastating to the most loving couples, even for those who have prepared for the possibility that they might fail. These are the times we advise couples to seek psychological counseling to help them cope with such painful losses. The counseling is usually short-term but intense and can be especially helpful in reestablishing a couple's sense of emotional equilibrium.

Counseling can be particularly effective in helping couples decide about the end of fertility treatments. Feeling depressed or anxious is a quite understandable response to this highly uncertain and emotionally painful time. Talking to someone about your feelings may help you move on to the next step in your lives together as a couple.

In the Future

Harvard researchers have shown that women who go through a mind-body program using cognitive behavioral therapy can get 40 percent higher pregnancy rates than those who don't participate in the program. Couples experience a high level of anxiety during most aspects of ART procedures. If researchers could understand the relationship between stress and anxiety and the release of stress hormones during ART procedures, they might be able to target specific variables and enhance the success of IVF.

An ongoing study at Weill Cornell is designed to do just that. We are looking carefully at ten biological markers and are using psychological testing to monitor several hundred first-time IVF patients. The women are tested when they first come in for treatment, before egg retrieval, and again after egg retrieval. The idea is to see if we can identify positive ways to help manage the inevitable stress of IVF and help more women have babies.

Take-Home Messages

- Feelings of depression, guilt, isolation, or anger are very common among infertile couples.
- The more you know about your condition, its causes, and treatments, the less stress you will feel about it.
- You can manage the effects of stress through techniques such as breathing exercises, journal writing, meditation and relaxation, mindfulness, and making time for yourself.
- You can learn to replace negative thoughts with new, more balanced thoughts.
- You and your partner may respond differently to infertility. Support each other and try to understand your partner's feelings.
- If family, friends, or strangers ask an insensitive question, have a rehearsed response ready to help you change the subject quickly.
- If you have secondary infertility, you may have feelings of guilt, denial, depression, and anxiety similar to someone who has primary infertility.
- Even if you have never been in counseling before, infertility could be the one reason to bring you to see a professional counselor. A wide variety of therapies can help you cope with infertility.
- If you are unable to conceive naturally, then you and your partner need to consider other options, such as donor embryo, donor egg, or adoption.

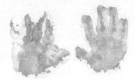

Conclusion

*N*ow that you've read through *A Baby At Last!* and are trying to conceive a child, we hope that you have elevated your understanding about the necessary steps required to achieve a pregnancy, how sperm and eggs meet, and what is needed for normal embryo implantation. This knowledge should give you insight into how we diagnose and treat infertility—from simple therapies to advanced reproductive technologies. It's our earnest hope that our straightforward approach to overcoming infertility will make it easier for you to attain your goal of having a baby at last.

Resources

Infertility Organizations

American Association of Tissue Banks
http://aatb.org
1320 Old Chain Bridge Road, Suite 450
McLean, VA 22101
(703) 827-9582
Supplies list of AATB-associated sperm
banks in the United States and Canada.

American Congress of Obstetricians and
Gynecologists Resource Center
http://www.acog.org/departments/dept
_web.cfm?recno=20
PO Box 96920
Washington, DC 20090-6920
(202) 638-5577
This national organization of obstetricians
and gynecologists has a resource center
that can provide patient education
pamphlets, lists of obstetricians and
gynecologists in regions of the country,
and answers to basic questions about
infertility and women's health.

American Fertility Association
http://afafamilymatters.com
305 Madison Avenue, Suite 449
New York, NY 10165
Support Line (888) 917-3777
This national nonprofit organization
is a resource for infertility prevention,
reproductive health, and family-building.
Services include an extensive online
library, monthly online Webinars, telephone
and in-person coaching, a resource

directory, an "Ask the Experts" online
feature, daily fertility news, and a toll-free
support line.

American Pregnancy Association
http://americanpregnancy.org
1431 Greenway Drive, Suite 800
Irving, Texas 75038
(972) 550-0140
This national health organization promotes
reproductive and pregnancy wellness
through education, research, advocacy, and
community awareness. It offers a general
overview of infertility and specific
information about alternative treatments
and reproductive technologies.

American Society for Reproductive
Medicine
http://www.asrm.org
1209 Montgomery Highway
Birmingham, AL 35216-2809
(205) 978-5000
The national organization of fertility
specialists provides general information
about infertility and patient pamphlets.

American Society of Andrology
http://andrologysociety.com
1100 E. Woodfield Road, Suite 520
Schaumburg, IL 60173
(847) 619-4909
Refers patients to andrologists across the
country.

American Urological Association
http://www.auanet.org
1000 Corporate Boulevard
Linthicum, MD 21090
Toll-free (U.S. only): (866) 746-4282
(410) 689-3700
Provides patient information pamphlets
and also supplies information about specific
questions and possible referrals to a local
urologist.

Endometriosis Association
http://endometriosisassn.org
8585 N. 76th Place
Milwaukee, WI 53223
(414) 355-2200
Furnishes a free brochure and general
information regarding endometriosis,
including local support groups and
education and research programs.

National Society of Genetic Counselors
http://www.nsgc.org
401 N. Michigan Avenue
Chicago, IL 60611
(312) 321-6834
Provides information on genetic counseling
services and referrals.

Planned Parenthood Federation of America
http://www.plannedparenthood.org
434 West 33rd Street
New York, NY 10001
(212) 541-7800
Provides referral to local Planned
Parenthood affiliates that may supply
infertility diagnosis and counseling.

Resolve: The National Infertility
Association
http://www.resolve.org
1760 Old Meadow Rd., Suite 500
McLean, VA 22102
(703) 556-7172

This national self-help group for infertile
couples provides physician and IVF referrals,
literature about many aspects of infertility, a
newsletter, and telephone counseling. It has
support groups across the country.

Internet Services

The Center for Reproductive Medicine
and Infertility
http://www.ivf.org
Dr. Rosenwaks's Web site

Center for Male Reproductive Medicine
and Microsurgery
http://www.maleinfertility.org
Dr. Goldstein's Web site

Centers for Disease Control (CDC)
Reproductive Health
http://www.cdc.gov/art/
This federal government Web site provides
success rates for all clinics that have
registered with the ASRM's Society for
Assisted Reproductive Technology.

The International Council on Infertility
Information Dissemination
(INCIID, pronounced "inside")
http://inciid.org
Inciid is "dedicated to helping infertile
couples explore their family-building
options, including treatment, adoption, and
choosing to live child-free." This site offers
both basic and advanced articles about
specific topics, dozens of fact sheets, bulletin
boards run by experts, and chat rooms.

Internet Health Resources
http://ihr.com
This business-to-consumer Web site offers
infertility education, services, and products,
with listings on a wide variety of topics
related to both female and male infertility.

About.com
http://pregnancy.about.com
The Pregnancy & Childbirth section has
information concerning infertility issues.
http://infertility.about.com
The Fertility section offers an overview
of infertility, plus fertility forums.

Fertility Plus
http://fertilityplus.org
This Web site offers information about
both beginning and advanced fertility
issues; infertility and related newsgroups,
list servers, bulletin boards, chat rooms,
and mail lists (for general infertility and
specific diagnoses); and resources for
donor sperm, donor egg, surrogacy, and
embryo adoption.

The Fertility Advocate
http://thefertilityadvocate.com/wpblog
Blog by Pamela Madsen, former Executive
Director of the American Fertility
Association

She Knows
http://talk.sheknows.com/
This Web site offers many message boards
for women to share information, including
the "Trying to Conceive Clubs."

Fertility Ties
http://fertilityties.com
This online community for fertility
patients offers information, support, tools,
and forums

IVF News.Direct!
http://ivfnewsdirect.com/
This Web site provides breaking news
about fertility for reproductive medicine
professionals and patients.

IVF-Infertility.com
http://ivf-infertility.com/
This Web site provides comprehensive
information about infertility as well as
specifics about IVF and ICSI. It also
offers a message board and chat forums.

Notes

Chapter 1: You Are Not Alone

6 *More than one third of all pregnancies and births in the United States:* B. E. Hamilton, J. A. Martin, and S. J. Ventura, "Births: Preliminary Data for 2006," *National Vital Statistics Reports* 56, no. 7 (2007).

9 *At age forty, the chances that a fetus will have Down syndrome:* March of Dimes, "Pregnancy after 35," Quick Reference Fact Sheet, http://www.marchofdimes.com/professionals/14332_1155.asp, accessed Jan. 1, 2009.

Chapter 2: What Factors Determine His Fertility?

17 *one of the consequences of diabetes:* I. M. Agbaje, D. A. Rogers, C. M. McVica, et al., "Insulin Dependant Diabetes Mellitus: Implications for Male Reproductive Function," *Human Reproduction* 22, no. 7 (2007): 1871–1877.

21 *paroxetine (Paxil), seems to increase DNA fragmentation:* C. Tanrikut, A. S. Feldman, M. Altemus, et al., "Adverse Effect of Paroxetine on Sperm," *Fertility and Sterility* (2009), published online June 10, 2009, at http://www.fertstert.org.

24 *Overweight men who have a body mass index:* R. H. Nguyen, A. J. Wilcox, R. Skjaerven, et al., "Men's Body Mass Index and Infertility," *Human Reproduction* 22, no. 9 (2007): 2488–2493.

29 *A range of pesticide classes has been investigated:* M. J. Perry, "Effects of Environmental and Occupational Pesticide Exposure on Human Sperm: A Systematic Review," *Human Reproduction Update* 14, no. 3 (2008): 233–242.

29 *Researchers at Nanjing Medical University:* Y. Xia, P. Zhu, Y. Han, et al., "Urinary Metabolites of Polycyclic Aromatic Hydrocarbons in Relation to Idiopathic Male Infertility," *Human Reproduction* 24, no. 5 (2009): 1067–1074.

30 *pregnant women who ate beef:* S. H. Swan, F. Liu, J. W. Overstreet, et al., "Semen Quality of Fertile U.S. Males in Relation to Their Mothers' Beef Consumption during Pregnancy," *Human Reproduction* 22 (2007): 1497–1502.

31 *large study of couples undergoing IUI:* S. Belloc, P. Cohen-Bacrie, M. Benkhalifa, et al., "Effect of Maternal and Paternal Age on Pregnancy and Miscarriage Rates after Intrauterine Insemination," *Reproductive Biomedicine Online* 17, no. 3 (2008): 392–397.

32 *association between cell phone use and sperm quality:* K. Makker, A. Varghese, N. R. Desai, et al., "Cell Phones: Modern Man's Nemesis?" *Reproductive Biomedicine Online* 18, no. 1 (2009): 148–157.

33 *higher levels of urinary BPA and poor semen quality:* S. Ehrlich, D. Wright, J. Ford, et al., "Urinary Bisphenol A Concentrations and Human Semen Quality," *Fertility and Sterility* 90 (2008): S186.

Chapter 3: What Factors Determine Her Fertility?

41 *heavy smokers (more than ten cigarettes a day):* S. R. Soares, C. Simon, J. Remohi, and A. Pellicer, "Cigarette Smoking Affects Uterine Receptiveness," *Human Reproduction* 22, no. 2 (2007): 543–547.

41 *secondhand smoke during both childhood* and *adulthood:* L. J. Peppone, K. M. Piazza, M. C. Mahoney, et al., "Associations between Adult and Childhood Secondhand Smoke Exposures and Fecundity and Fetal Loss among Women Who Visited a Cancer Hospital," *Tobacco Control* 18 (2009): 115–120.

42 *women exposed to sidestream smoke:* M. S. Neal, E. G. Hughes, A. C. Holloway, and W. G. Foster, "Sidestream Smoking Is Equally as Damaging as Mainstream Smoking on IVF Outcomes," *Human Reproduction* 20, no. 9 (2005): 2531–2551.

42 *the higher the BMI in obese women:* J. W. van der Steeg, P. Steures, M. J. Eijkemans, et al., "Obesity Affects Spontaneous Pregnancy Chances in Subfertile Ovulatory Women," *Human Reproduction* 23, no. 2 (2008): 324–328.

43 *genetic connection between obesity and PCOS:* T. M. Barber, A. J. Bennett, C. J. Groves, et al., "Association of Variants within the Fat Mass and Obesity-Associated (FTO) Gene and Polycystic Ovary Syndrome," *Diabetologia* 51, no. 7 (2008): 1153–1158.

43 *alterations in the fluid bathing the eggs:* R. L. Robker, L. K. Akison, B. D. Bennett, et al., "Obese Women Exhibit Differences in Ovarian Metabolites, Hormones, and Gene Expression Compared with Moderate-Weight Women," *Journal of Clinical Endocrinology and Metabolism* 94, no. 5 (2009): 1533–1540.

43 *BMI seems to have a significant negative impact:* M. L. Sneed, M. L. Uhler, H. E. Grotjan, et al., "Body Mass Index Impact on IVF Success Appears Age Related," *Human Reproduction* 23, no. 8 (2008): 1835–1839.

44 *cortisol can affect this hormone cascade:* O. B. Damti, O. Sarid, and E. Sheiner, "Stress and Distress in Infertility among Women," *Harefuah* 147, no 3 (2008): 256–260, 276.

44 *women who consumed two alcoholic drinks per day:* J. Eggert, H. Theobald, and P. Engfeldt, "Effects of Alcohol Consumption on Female Fertility during an 18-Year Period," *Fertility and Sterility* 81, no. 2 (2004): 379–383.

45 *Even moderate amounts of caffeine:* A. Wilcox, C. Weinberg, and D. Baird, "Caffeinated Beverages and Decreased Fertility," *Lancet* 2, no. 8626–8627 (1988): 1453–1456.

46 *Exposure to the 87,000 chemicals in commercial use:* T. J. Woodruff, A. Carlson, J. M. Schwartz, et al., "Proceedings of the Summit on Environmental Challenges to Reproductive Health and Fertility: Executive Summary," *Fertility and Sterility* 89, no. 2 (2008): 281–300.

46 *farm or greenhouse workers, may be less likely to conceive:* L. Lauria, "Exposure to Pesticides and Time to Pregnancy among Female Greenhouse Workers," *Reproductive Toxicology* 22, no. 3 (2006): 425–430.

46 *women who have used pesticides in their homes:* K. G. Harley, A. R. Marks, A. Bradman, et al., "DDT Exposure, Work in Agriculture and Time to Pregnancy among Farmworkers in California," *Journal of Occupational and Environmental Medicine* 50, no. 12 (2008): 1335–1342.

46 *heavy metals, particularly lead, interferes:* P. Mendola, L. C. Messer, K. Rappazzo, "Science Linking Environmental Contaminant Exposures with Fertility and Reproductive Health Impacts in the Adult Female," *Fertility and Sterility* 89, no. 2, Suppl. (2008): e81–e94.

47 *PFCs may interfere with hormones that are involved in reproduction:* T. I. Halldorsson,

C. Fei, J. Olsen, et al., "Dietary Predictors of Perfluorinated Chemicals: A Study from the Danish National Birth Cohort," *Environmental Science and Technology* 42, no. 23 (2008): 8971–8977.

48 *has also been associated with PCOS:* D. A. Crain, S. J. Janssen, T. M. Edwards, et al., "Female Reproductive Disorders: The Roles of Endocrine-Disrupting Compounds and Developmental Timing," *Fertility and Sterility* 90, no.4 (2008): 911–940.

Chapter 4: What a Couple Can Do

51 *practicing relaxation techniques regularly:* T. M. Cousineau and A. D. Domar, "Psychological Impact of Infertility," *Best Practice and Research Clinical Obstetrics and Gynaecology* 21, no. 2 (2007): 293–308.

53 *if they lose weight, their sex hormone levels will likely improve:* A. Hammoud, M. Gibson, S. C. Hunt, et al., "Effect of Roux-en-Y Gastric Bypass Surgery on the Sex Steroids and Quality of Life in Obese Men," *Journal of Clinical Endocrinology and Metabolism* 94, no. 4 (2009): 1329–1332.

54 *the more fresh produce a man eats, the more active his sperm:* V. Lewis, L. Kochman, R. Herko, "Dietary Antioxidants and Sperm Quality in Infertile Men," *Fertility and Sterility* 86, no. 3 (2006): S364–S364.

62 *men who consumed the most folate:* S. S. Young, B. Eskenazi, F. M. Marchetti, et al., "The Association of Folate, Zinc and Antioxidant Intake with Sperm Aneuploidy in Healthy Non-Smoking Men," *Human Reproduction* 23, no. 5 (2008): 1014–1022.

62 *men who consumed half a serving of soy foods each day:* J. E. Chavarro, T. L. Toth, S. M. Sadio, et al., "Soy Food and Isoflavone Intake in Relation to Semen Quality Parameters among Men from an Infertility Clinic," *Human Reproduction* 23, no. 11 (2008): 2584–2590.

63 *what you eat and drink can impact the reproductive system:* J. E. Chavarro, J. W. Rich-Edwards, B. A. Rosner, et al., "Diet and Lifestyle in the Prevention of Ovulatory Disorder Infertility," *Obstetrics and Gynecology* 110, no. 5 (2007): 1050–1058.

Chapter 5: Who's on Your Team?

67 *Male-factor infertility is mentioned on less than two thirds:* D. H. Williams and J. D. Nelson, "The Use of Biased Language and Inaccurate Information about Male Factor Infertility on Fertility Clinic Websites in the United States," *Fertility and Sterility* 90, Suppl. (2008): S3.

Chapter 6: What Tests Should a Man Have?

83 *men with infertility and abnormal sperm counts:* J. D. Raman, C. F. Nobert, and M. Goldstein, "Increased Incidence of Testicular Cancer in Men Presenting with Infertility and Abnormal Semen Analysis," *Journal of Urology* 174 (2005): 1819–1822; and T. J. Walsh, M. S. Croughan, M. Schembri, et al., "Increased Risk of Testicular Germ Cell Cancer among Infertile Men," *Archives of Internal Medicine* 169, no. 4(2009): 351–356.

89 *men with large varicoceles have lower sperm counts:* J. Steckel, A. P. Dicker, and M. Goldstein, "Influence of Varicocele Size on Response to Microsurgical Ligation of the Spermatic Veins," *Journal of Urology* 149(1993): 769–771.

89 *varicoceles raise the temperature inside the testicles:* M. Goldstein and J. F. Eid, "Elevation of Intratesticular and Scrotal Skin Surface Temperature in Men with Varicocele," *Journal of Urology* 142(1989): 743–745; and E. J. Wright, G. P. H. Young, and M. Goldstein, "Reduction in Testicular Temperature after Varicocelectomy in Infertile Men," *Urology* 50 (1997): 257–259.

Chapter 7: What Tests Should a Woman Have?

101 *cause malformations in the reproductive organs:* S. H. Swan, "Intrauterine Exposure to Diethylstilbestrol: Long-Term Effects in Humans. Review Article," *Acta Pathologica, Microbiologica et Immunologica Scandinavica* 108 (2000): 793–804.

Chapter 8: Taking Action for Men

116 *most urologists who perform varicocele repairs:* S. S. Sehgal, D. I. Chu, B. J. Otto, et al., "Survey of Varicocelectomy Techniques Employed by AUA Urologists," *Journal of Urology* 179, no. 4 (2008): 657.

117 *following varicocele repair, testosterone levels are greatly improved:* L. M. Su, M. Goldstein, and P. N. Schlegel, "The Effect of Varicocelectomy on Serum Testosterone Levels in Infertile Men with Varicoceles," *Journal of Urology* 154, no. 5 (1995): 1752–1755.

128 *Color Doppler ultrasound is proving somewhat predictive:* M. Cocuzza, R. Pagani, R. Coelho, et al., "The Systematic Use of Intraoperative Vascular Doppler Ultrasound during Microsurgical Subinguinal Varicocelectomy Improves Precise Identification and Preservation of Testicular Blood Supply," *Fertility and Sterility* (2009), published online March 6, 2009, at http://www.fertstert.org.

129 *two drugs extended the time to orgasm:* M. Wyllie, P. Heath, and W. Dinsmore, "PSD502, a Novel Metered-Dose Aerosol Formulation of Lidocaine and Prilocaine, Is a Safe and Effective Treatment for Premature Ejaculation (PE); Results of a Phase III, Randomized, Double-Blind, Placebo-Controlled Study," *Journal of Urology* 181, no. 4 (2009): 489. References and further reading may be available with purchase of this article.

Chapter 9: Taking Action for Women

136 *an increased risk of ovarian cancer:* A. Jensen, H. Sharif, and K. Frederiksen, "Use of Fertility Drugs and Risk of Ovarian Cancer: Danish Population Based Cohort Study," *British Medical Journal* 338 (2009): b249.

146 *kisspeptin injections showed marked increases in their blood levels:* C. N. Jayasena and W. S. Dhillo, "Kisspeptin Offers a Novel Therapeutic Target in Reproduction," *Current Opinion in Investigational Drugs* 10, no. 4 (2009): 311–318.

Chapter 10: Am I a Candidate for IVF?

158 *IVF does not increase the risk of developmental disorders:* K. J. Middelburg, M. L. Haadsma, M. J. Heineman, et al., "Ovarian Hyperstimulation and the In Vitro Fertilization Procedure Do Not Influence Early Neuromotor Development, a History of Subfertility Does," *Fertility and Sterility* (2009), published online April 9, 2009, at http://www.fertstert.org.

158 *IVF kids may grow taller:* H. L. Miles, P. L. Hofman, J. Peek, et al., "In Vitro Fertilization Improves Childhood Growth and Metabolism," *Journal of Clinical Endocrinology and Metabolism* 92, no. 9 (2007): 3441–3445.

161 *couples with full insurance coverage are more willing to try:* R. J. Stillman, K. S. Richter, N. K. Banks, et al., "Elective Single Embryo Transfer: A 6-Year Progressive Implementation of 784 Single Blastocyst Transfers and the Influence of Payment Method on Patient Choice," *Fertility and Sterility* 92, no. 6 (2009): 1895–1906.

164 *success rates are much lower for those over forty:* B. A. Malizia, M. Hacker, and A. Penzias, "Cumulative Live-Birth Rates after In Vitro Fertilization," *New England Journal of Medicine* 360, no. 3 (2009): 236–243.

166 *frozen embryos are healthier than fresh embryos:* A. Pinborg, A. Loft, A. K. Aaris Henningsen, et al., "Infant Outcome of 957 Singletons Born after Frozen Embryo Replacement: The Danish National Cohort Study 1995–2006," *Fertility and Sterility* (2009), published online July 31, 2009, at http://www.fertstert.org.

167 *called* karyomapping, *analyzes chromosomes:* A. Handyside, N. Zech, B. Mariani, et al., "Genome Wide Karyomapping for Preimplantation Genetic Diagnosis (PGD) Detects Inherited Chromosomal Aneuploidies," *Fertility and Sterility* 92, no. 3 (2009): S204.

167 *physiology of an embryo using metabolomic profiling:* L. Botros, D. Sakkas, and E. Seli, 167Metabolomics and Its Application for Noninvasive Embryo Assessment in IVF," *Molecular Human Reproduction* 14, no. 12 (2008): 679–690.

Chapter 11: Am I a Candidate for ICSI?

172 *embryos that form from ICSI are just as healthy:* Q. V. Neri, T. Takeuchi, and G. D. Palermo, "An Update of Assisted Reproductive Technologies Results in the United States," *Annals of New York Academy of Sciences* 1127 (2008): 41–48.

173 *For the nearly ten thousand couples we have treated:* G. D. Palermo, Q. V. Neri, T. Takeuchi, et al., "ICSI: Where We Have Been and Where We Are Going," *Seminars in Reproductive Medicine* 27, no. 2 (2009): 191–201.

174 *no problems in terms of psychological or physical development:* I. Ponjaert-Kristoffersen, T. Tjus, J. Nekkebroeck, et al., on behalf of the Collaborative Study of Brussels, Göteborg, and New York, "Psychological Follow-Up Study of 5-Year-Old ICSI Children," *Human Reproduction* 19, no. 12 (2004): 2791–2797.

174 *early development of the children born using ICSI:* G. D. Palermo, Q. V. Neri, T. Takeuchi, et al., "Genetic and Epigenetic Characteristics of ICSI Children," *Reproductive Biomedicine Online* 17, no. 6 (2008): 820–833.

178 *never have been able to become biological fathers:* R. Ramasamy, J. A. Ricci, G. D. Palermo, et al., "Successful Fertility Treatment for Klinefelter's Syndrome," *Journal of Urology* 182, no. 3 (2009): 1108–1113.

180 *examine the quality of a sperm without damaging it:* T. Huser, C. A. Orme, C. W. Hollars, et al., "Raman Spectroscopy of DNA Packaging in Individual Human Sperm Cells Distinguishes Normal from Abnormal Cells," *Journal of Biophotonics* 2, no. 5 (2009): 322–332.

180 *chances of the woman miscarrying may be higher:* A. Zini, J. M. Boman, E. Belzile, et al., "Sperm DNA Damage Is Associated with an Increased Risk of Pregnancy Loss after IVF and ICSI: Systematic Review and Meta-Analysis," *Human Reproduction* 23, no. 12 (2008): 2663–2668.

Chapter 12: What Are My Other Options?

186 *Repeated attempts at IVF with endometrial-cell co-culture:* S. D. Spandorfer, R. Clark, J. Park, et al., "Autologous Endometrial Co-Culture (AECC): An Effective Tool for Patients with Multiple Failed IVF Attempts," *Fertility and Sterility* 80, no. 3 (2003): 6.

192 *PGD testing allows parents to make choices:* S. Baruch, "Preimplantation Genetic Diagnosis and Parental Preferences: Beyond Deadly Disease," *Houston Journal of Health Law and Policy* 8 (2008): 245–270.

192 *most people would elect to have prenatal genetic testing:* F. Hathaway, E. Burns, and H. Ostrer, "Consumer's Desire towards Current and Prospective Reproductive Genetic Testing," *Journal of Genetic Counseling* 18, no. 2 (2009): 137–146.

193 *identify the best embryos to transfer:* G. M. Jones, D. S. Cram, B. Song, et al., "Novel Strategy with Potential to Identify Developmentally Competent IVF Blastocysts," *Human Reproduction* 23, no. 8 (2008): 1748–1759.

194 *use the three genetic markers to select eggs:* Y. Guillemin, P. Lalle, G. Gillet, et al., "Oocytes and Early Embryos Selectively Express the Survival Factor BCL2L10," *Journal of Molecular Medicine* 87, no. 9 (2009): 923–940.

Chapter 13: Third-Party Reproduction

199 *fewer than 1 percent of the egg donors had serious complications:* K. N. Maxwell, I. N. Cholst, and Z. Rosenwaks, "The Incidence of Both Serious and Minor Complications in Young Women Undergoing Oocyte Donation," *Fertility and Sterility* 90, no. 6 (2008): 2165–2171.

201 *the egg donor's time and commitment:* S. Covington and W. Gibbons, "What Is Happening to the Price of Eggs?" *Fertility and Sterility* 87, no. 5 (2007): 1001–1004.

201 *women who donate eggs primarily for altruistic reasons:* N. J. Kenney and M. L. McGowan, "Looking Back: Egg Donors' Retrospective Evaluations of Their Motivations, Expectations, and Experiences during Their First Donation Cycle," *Fertility and Sterility* (2008), published online November 19, 2008, at http://www.fertstert.org.

208 *genes that cause premature ovarian failure:* H. Zhao, Z.-J. Chen, Y. Qin, et al., "Transcription Factor FIGLA Is Mutated in Patients with Premature Ovarian Failure," *American Journal of Human Genetics* 82, no. 6 (2008): 1342–1348.

209 *function of these genetic variants in early menopause:* L. Stolk, G. Zhai, J. B. van Meurs, et al., "Loci at Chromosomes 13, 19 and 20 Influence Age at Natural Menopause," *Nature Genetics* 41 (2009): 645–647.

Chapter 14: Other Fertility Issues

213 *a method called cell reprogramming:* J. Yu, M. A. Vodyanik, K. Smuga-Otto, et al., "Induced Pluripotent Stem Cell Lines Derived from Human Somatic Cells," *Science* 318, no. 5858 (2007): 1917–1920; and K. Okita, T. Ichisaka, and S. Yamanaka, "Generation of Germline-Competent Induced Pluripotent Stem Cells," *Nature* 448, no. 7151 (2007): 313–317.

213 *relieved Parkinson disease symptoms in rats:* M. Wernig, J. P. Zhao, J. Pruszak, et al., "Neurons Derived from Reprogrammed Fibroblasts Functionally Integrate into the Fetal Brain and Improve Symptoms of Rats with Parkinson's Disease," *Proceedings of the National Academy of Sciences* 105, no. 15 (2008): 5856–5861.

213 *human skin cells of Parkinson disease patients:* F. Soldner, D. Hockemeyer, and C. Beard, "Parkinson's Disease Patient-Derived Induced Pluripotent Stem Cells Free of Viral Reprogramming Factors," *Cell* 136, no. 5 (2009): 964–977.

213 *stem cells in the laboratory from adult cells:* H. Zhou, S. Wu, J. Y. Joo, et al., "Generation of Induced Pluripotent Stem Cells Using Recombinant Proteins," *Cell Stem Cell* 4, no. 5 (2009): 381–384.

214 *reprogrammed blood cells to act as embryonic stem cells:* Y. H. Loh, S. Agarwal, I. H. Park, et al., "Generation of Induced Pluripotent Stem Cells from Human Blood," *Blood* 113, no. 22 (2009): 5476–5479.

214 *early spermatogonia (sperm-forming cells):* M. Seandel, D. James, S. V. Shmelkov, et al., "Generation of Functional Multipotent Adult Stem Cells from GPR125+ Germline Progenitors," *Nature* 449, no. 7160 (2007): 346–350.

215 *spermlike cells into two hundred mouse eggs:* G. D. Palermo, Q. V. Neri, T. Takeuchi, et al., "ICSI: Where We Have Been and Where We Are Going," *Seminars in Reproductive Medicine* 27, no. 2 (2009): 191–201.

216 *extracted stem cells from the testicles of men:* S. Conrad, M. Renninger, J. Hennenlotter, et al., "Generation of Pluripotent Stem Cells from Adult Human Testis," *Nature* 456, no. 7220 (2008): 344–349; N. Golestaneh, M. Kokkinaki, D. Pant, et al., "Pluripotent Stem Cells Derived from Adult Human Testes," *Stem Cells and Development* 18, no. 8 (2009): 1115–1126; and N. Kossack, J. Meneses, S. Shefi, et al., "Isolation and Characterization of Pluripotent Human Spermatogonial Stem Cell-Derived Cells," *Stem Cells* 27, no. 1 (2009): 138–149.

217 *donate the embryos for stem-cell research:* A. D. Lyerly, K. Steinhauser, C. Voils, et al., "Fertility Patients' Views about Frozen Embryo Disposition: Results of a Multi-Institutional U.S. Survey," *Fertility and Sterility* (2008), published online December 5, 2008, at http://www.fertstert.org.

217 *not morally wrong to use embryonic stem cells:* T. Jain and S. A. Missmer, "Support for Embryonic Stem Cell Research among Infertility Patients," *Fertility and Sterility* 90, no. 3 (2008): 506–512.

218 *cells that normally give rise to eggs:* K. Zou, Z. Yuan, Z. Yang, et al., "Production of Offspring from a Germline Stem Cell Line Derived from Neonatal Ovaries," *Nature Cell Biology* 11, no. 5 (2009): 631–636.

Chapter 15: Can We Still Get Pregnant after Cancer?

224 *create an embryo from banked frozen ovarian tissue:* K. Oktay, E. Buyuk, L. Veeck, et al., "Embryo Development after Heterotopic Transplantation of Cryopreserved Ovarian Tissue," *Lancet* 363, no. 9412 (2004): 837–840.

225 *Ovarian tissue freezing has become an option:* J. Donnez, B. Martinez-Madrid, P. Jadoul, et al., "Ovarian Tissue Cryopreservation and Transplantation: A Review," *Human Reproductive Update* 12, no. 5 (2006): 519–535.

226 *implanted a woman's entire ovary:* S. J. Silbert, G. Grudzinskas, R. G. Gosden, "Successful Pregnancy after Microsurgical Transplantation of an Intact Ovary," *New England Journal of Medicine* 359, no. 24 (2008): 2617–2618.

229 *To remove a testicular tumor and preserve the testicle's function:* C. V. Hopps and M. Goldstein, "Ultrasound Guided Needle Localization and Microsurgical Exploration for Incidental Non-Palpable Testicular Tumors," *Journal of Urology* 168 (2002): 1084–1087.

229 *extract sperm from the normal tissue:* B. B. Choi, M. Goldstein, M. Moomjy, et al., "Births Using Sperm Retrieved via Immediate Micodissection of a Solitary Testis with Cancer," *Fertility and Sterility* 84, no. 5 (2005): 1508.e1–1508.e4.

230 *the male partner underwent chemo- or radiotherapy:* A. Hourvitz, D. E. Goldschlag, O. K. Davis, et al., "Intracytoplasmic Sperm Injection (ICSI) Using Cryopreserved Sperm from Men with Malignant Neoplasm Yields High Pregnancy Rates," *Fertility and Sterility* 90, no. 3 (2008): 557–563.

232 *many oncologists do not adequately address fertility issues:* G. Quinn, S. T. Vadaparampil, P. Jacobsen, et al., "National Survey of Physicians Practice Patterns: Fertility Preservation and Cancer Patients," *Journal of Clinical Oncology* 27, no. 18s (2009): CRA9508.

232 *how to preserve fertility in cancer patients:* S. J. Lee, ASCO Fertility Preservation Guidelines Committee, Z. Blumenfeld, K. Oktay, et al., "Preservation of Fertility in Patients with Cancer," *New England Journal of Medicine* 360, no. 25 (2009): 2680–2681.

233 *follicles from young female cancer patients:* M. Xu, S. L. Barrett, E. West-Farrell, et al., "In Vitro Grown Human Ovarian Follicles from Cancer Patients Support Oocyte Growth," *Human Reproduction* 24, no. 10 (2009): 2531–2540.

233 *retrieved, matured, and froze eggs from that tissue:* A. Revel, S. Revel-Vilk, E. Aizenman, et al., "At What Age Can Human Oocytes Be Obtained?" *Fertility and Sterility* 92, no. 2 (2009): 458–463.

Chapter 16: Do Alternative Treatments Work?

237 *reviewed recent studies of TCM in fertility:* S.-T. Huang and A. P.-C. Chen, "Traditional Chinese Medicine and Infertility," *Current Opinion in Obstetrics and Gynecology* 20, no. 3 (2008): 211–215.

238 *acupuncture treatments and increased production of endorphins:* R. Chang, P. H. Chung, and Z. Rosenwaks, "Role of Acupuncture in the Treatment of Female Infertility," *Fertility and Sterility* 78, no. 6 (2002): 1149–1153.

239 *study by researchers at the University of Ulm:* W. E. Paulus, M. Zhang, E. Strehler, et al., "Influence of Acupuncture on the Pregnancy Rate in Patients Who Undergo Assisted Reproduction Therapy," *Fertility and Sterility* 77, no. 4 (2002): 721–724.

239 *acupuncture might improve the odds of conceiving:* E. Manheimer, G. Zhang, L. Udoff, et al., "Effects of Acupuncture on Rates of Pregnancy and Live Birth among Women Undergoing in Vitro Fertilisation: Systematic Review and Meta-Analysis," *British Medical Journal* 336, no. 7643 (2008): 545–549.

240 *acupuncture may not improve IVF success rates:* T. El-Toukhy and Y. Khalaf, "The Impact of Acupuncture on Assisted Reproductive Technology Outcome," *Current Opinion in Obstetrics and Gynecology* 21, no. 3 (2009): 240–246.

240 *they were less anxious after the embryo transfer:* A. D. Domar, I. Meshay, J. Kelliher, et al., "The Impact of Acupuncture on In Vitro Fertilization Outcome," *Fertility and Sterility* 91, no. 3 (2009): 723–726.

240 *Cochrane Collaboration review of data:* Y. C. Cheong, E. Hung Yu Ng, and W. L. Ledger, "Acupuncture and Assisted Conception," *Cochrane Database of Systematic Reviews* 4 (2008): CD006920.

241 *placebo acupuncture given on the day of embryo transfer:* E. W. So, E. H. Ng, Y. Y. Wong, et al., "A Randomized Double Blind Comparison of Real and Placebo Acupuncture in IVF Treatment," *Human Reproduction* 24, no. 2 (2009): 341–348.

242 *herbs act as antioxidants as well as antiestrogens:* H. G. Tempest, S. T. Homa, E. J. Routledge, et al., "Plants Used in Chinese Medicine for the Treatment of Male Infertility Possess Antioxidant and Anti-Oestrogenic Activity," *Systems Biology in Reproductive Medicine* 54, no. 4–5 (2008): 185–195.

243 *A pine tree bark extract:* S. J. Roseff, "Improvement in Sperm Quality and Function with French Maritime Pine Tree Bark Extract," *Journal of Reproductive Medicine* 47, no. 10 (2002): 821–824.

244 *if they had less stress in their lives:* S. M. S. Ebbesen, R. Zachariae, M. Y. Mehlsen, et al., "Stressful Life Events Are Associated with a Poor In-Vitro Fertilization IVF Outcome: A Prospective Study," *Human Reproduction* 24, no. 9 (2009): 2173–2182.

245 *psychosocial and medical profiles of 818 Danish women:* J. Boivin and L. Schmidt, "Infertility-Related Stress in Men and Women Predicts Treatment Outcome 1 Year Later," *Fertility and Sterility* 83, no. 6 (2005): 1745–1752.

247 *laser acupuncture treatments before and after embryo transfer:* J. L. Fratterelli, M. R. Leondires, K. Fong, et al., "Laser Acupuncture Before and After Embryo Transfer Improves ART Delivery Rates: Results of a Prospective Randomized Double-Blinded Placebo Controlled Five-Armed Trial Involving 1000 Patients," *Fertility and Sterility* 90, Suppl. (2008): S105.

Chapter 17: What About the Rest of My Life?

255 *women tend to experience greater levels of distress:* J. Wright, C. Duchesne, S. Sabourin, et al., "Psychosocial Distress and Infertility: Men and Women Respond Differently," *Fertility and Sterility* 55, no. 1 (1991): 100–108.

255 *depression or reduced quality of life in men:* A. Shindel, C. Nelson, C. Naughton, et al., "Sexual Function and Quality of Life in the Male Partner of Infertile Couples: Prevalence and Correlates of Dysfunction," *Journal of Urology* 179, no. 3 (2008): 1056–1059.

256 *men felt mental and physical stress:* L. A. Peronace, J. Boivin, and L. Schmidt, "Patterns of Suffering and Social Interactions in Infertile Men: 12 Months after Unsuccessful Treatment," *Journal of Psychosomatic Obstetrics and Gynecology* 28, no. 2 (2007): 105–114.

256 *men who actively confronted their infertility:* L. Schmidt, B. Holstein, U. Christensen, et al., "Does Infertility Cause Marital Benefit: An Epidemiological Study of 2,250 Women and Men in Fertility Treatment," *Patient Education and Counseling* 59, no. 3 (2005): 244–251.

262 *women who go through a mind-body program:* A. D. Domar, M. M. Seibel, and H. Benson, "The Mind Body Program for Infertility: A New Behavioral Treatment Approach for Women with Infertility," *Fertility and Sterility* 53, no. 2 (1990): 246–249.

Index

ZEV ROSENWAKS, M.D., is the director and physician-in-chief of the Ronald O. Perelman and Claudia Cohen Center for Reproductive Medicine at the New York–Presbyterian Hospital/Weill Cornell Medical Center. He is also the Revlon Distinguished Professor of Reproductive Medicine in Obstetrics and Gynecology and professor of obstetrics and gynecology and reproductive medicine at Weill Cornell Medical College of Cornell University.

MARC GOLDSTEIN, M.D., is director of the Center for Male Reproductive Medicine and Microsurgery and surgeon-in-chief of male reproductive medicine and surgery at New York–Presbyterian Hospital/Weill Cornell Medical Center. He is also the Matthew P. Hardy Distinguished Professor of Reproductive Medicine and Urology at Weill Cornell Medical College of Cornell University.

MARK L. FUERST (www.marklfuerst.com) is a health and medical writer and the coauthor of nine books. He has been a freelance journalist for more than thirty years, and his articles have appeared in popular consumer magazines such as *Family Circle*, *Woman's Day*, *Health*, *Parents*, and *Self*. His articles on fertility have appeared in *Good Housekeeping*, *Woman's World*, *Baby Talk*, and publications of the United Features newspaper syndicate. As a staff writer for *Medical World News*, he wrote many articles and covered major medical meetings concerning fertility.

Mr. Fuerst earned a biology degree from Dickinson College and a master's degree in journalism from the University of Missouri at Columbia. He has been a member of the National Association of Science Writers for thirty years and for more than twenty-five years a member of the American Society of Journalists and Authors, for which he served as president from 1992 to 1994. He lives in Brooklyn, N.Y., with his wife and two children.